PRAISE FOR *VEGAN LUNCH BOX*

"Jennifer McCann's cookbook makes vegan cooking accessible and fun. It's informative but not stuffy, detailed yet concise, and the recipes are creative without being difficult. There are so many delicious, well put together options here, it's not only perfect for kids but for anyone who ever eats lunch!"

—Isa Chandra Moskowitz, author of *VEGANOMICON*

"Being a vegan kid just got a lot easier! The menus in *Vegan Lunch Box* make it easy to plan a balanced and nutritious lunch for your kids (or yourself!). The variety alone makes it worth having."

—Erin Pavlina, author of
RAISING VEGAN CHILDREN IN A NON-VEGAN WORLD

"Destined to become a classic, this is the book vegan parents have been waiting for. And who knew? A vegan mom started a blog describing the lunches she made for her son for one school year, and it won the 2006 Bloggie Award for "Best Food Blog" (NOT "best VEGETARIAN food blog," but "Best Food Blog," period!). It inspired, delighted, and motivated not only vegan parents, but omnivores bored with their own lackluster lunches. This book will continue delighting with recipes that are as innovative, kid-pleasing, and healthful as they are delicious."

—Bryanna Clark Grogan, author of *NONNA'S ITALIAN KITCHEN*

Vegan
Lunch Box

Vegan Lunch Box

150 Amazing, Animal-Free Lunches Kids and Grown-Ups Will Love!

Jennifer McCann

Da Capo

LIFE
LONG

A Member of the Perseus Books Group

Photographs © Greg McCann

Designed by Trish Wilkinson
Set in 12 point Goudy by the Perseus Books Group

Library of Congress Cataloging-in-Publication Data
McCann, Jennifer.
    Vegan lunch box : 150 amazing, animal-free lunches kids and grown-ups
will love! / Jennifer McCann. — 1st Da Capo Press ed.
        p.   cm.
    Includes index.
    ISBN 978-1-60094-072-9 (alk. paper)
    1. Vegan cookery. 2. Lunchbox cookery. I. Title.
TX837.M463 2008
641.5'636—dc22   2008004700

First Da Capo Press edition 2008

Published by Da Capo Press
A Member of the Perseus Books Group
www.dacapopress.com

Da Capo Press books are available at special discounts for bulk
purchases in the United States by corporations, institutions,
and other organizations. For more information, please contact the
Special Markets Department at the Perseus Books Group, 2300 Chestnut Street,
Suite 200, Philadelphia, PA 19103, or call (800) 810-4145, extension 5000,
or e-mail special.markets@perseusbooks.com.

1 2 3 4 5 6 7 8 9

"Give children a healthy dose of the truth, and I believe most of them will hop, skip, and jump over to the side of the angels and never look back."

Howard Lyman, *NO MORE BULL!*

Acknowledgments

THANKS . . .

To all the visitors to the Vegan Lunch Box blog—everyone who left behind a kind word, voted for me, tested recipes, and asked me to be their mom (okay, now go clean your room).

To my friends Elizabeth Schroeder, Linda Frederick, and Chelee Ellis for recipe testing; Martie Sahuc for inspiring me with her story; Joshua Ploeg for the Satya gig; Renee Pottle for your wisdom, help, and inspiration. To Dione Ruff-Sloan, Tina Stephenson, Amy Nylund, and Candace d'Obrenovic for their contributions.

To Erik Marcus, Erin Pavlina, and Dreena Burton, for your mentoring and advice, and for all the vital work you do. To PETA for the Proggy Award and VegNews for the Veg Webby Award.

Very special thanks to Diane Molleson for all her help.

To my whole family: with love to my husband, Greg, for his photography, advice, support, encouragement, and for putting up with me; to my mom, Susan Moore, for teaching me to cook with love, and to Ted Moore for all the asparagus; to my dad, David Andrews, for desert hikes and Adobe advice, and to Wilma Andrews for her spirit; to my aunt, Julie Adamson, for teaching me to love sushi; and to my sister-in-law Rachel Andrews, for stuffed peppers and recipe testing.

. . . and most of all, to my son, James Henry. Thanks for being such a good eater.

Contents

Part Two
THE RECIPES

Foreword by Erik Marcus

No matter how good a mother's intentions, it will often seem that the world doesn't want children to be vegan. From birthday parties to day camp outings, being a child in America means being offered animal products dozens of times each year. And of all the hazards facing the vegan child, none compares to what happens every day during the school lunch period.

School cafeterias are enemy territory to vegetarian and vegan kids. Nearly all these cafeterias serve as the dumping grounds for the commodity meat and dairy products purchased by the USDA's price support program. What's worse, meat industry lobbyists have succeeded in shaping the National School Lunch Program's nutritional guidelines, so that protein requirements and saturated fat allowances are kept unreasonably high. In consequence, most school cafeterias serve meals that resemble some Frankensteinian mishmash of all the worst foods McDonald's, Taco Bell, and Long John Silver's have to offer. Breaded nuggets and french fries, anyone?

This insanely unhealthy system seems destined to crumble within the next generation, but that's little comfort to vegan mothers whose children are starting school today. It was in exactly this situation that Jennifer McCann found herself back in 2005. Her seven-year-old son, James, was starting the first grade. Soon, every afternoon, he would find himself in the school cafeteria watching his friends and classmates devour cheeseburgers, pizza, and fried chicken. What could Jennifer send her son to school with each day that would ensure he wouldn't feel tempted to eat like the other kids?

The answer: give James a lunch that is better—much better—than anything served to his classmates. And by better, I don't simply mean healthier—I mean better in every respect. Every school day, Jennifer cooks up a miniature four-course meal that trumps the cafeteria's offerings in terms of flavor, color, texture, creativity, and especially love. She packages these meals in snazzy, Japanese-style bento lunchboxes and also frequently relies on a Thermos for soups, sauces, and cold drinks.

Every mother must worry that, by not eating like other kids, their children will be isolated and even ridiculed for their diet. But James's lunches have made him anything but a pariah. His classmates know great-looking food when they see it, and so his lunches have made James the envy of his school.

Appreciation for James's lunches extends well beyond the walls of his cafeteria. In 2005, Jennifer started her blog at veganlunchbox .com. And with that, James has become not just the envy of his fellow first graders but the poster boy for an international audience of thousands of kids, parents, and other lovers of great food. Each school day, Jennifer posts a photo of her latest offering, complete with write-up, cooking summary, and notes on what James ate, didn't eat, loved, hated, or merely tolerated. Based on James's evaluations, Jennifer awards each meal from one to five stars. Every recipe in this book has been rated five stars—certification of absolute James approval.

If it sounds like, over the course of each school year, James samples hundreds of different foods, well, that's absolutely correct. Where a typical seven-year-old might think a corn dog exemplifies gourmet creativity, little James has already experienced vastly more foods than a typical American eats in an entire lifetime. He's dined on Mexican flautas, Japanese vegan sushi, Irish stew, and a seemingly unending variety of other foods. As you can see, James has absolutely no cause to feel left out when the lunch bell rings each day—rather, it's his classmates who are envious.

James's lunches help to illustrate exactly what's gone wrong with the National School Lunch Program, and how this dire situation could quickly be remedied. We would never tolerate an elementary school that failed to teach its students to read, to add and subtract, and to know something of history and geography. But in most American schools, the learning stops when the lunch bell rings. Upon shuffling into the cafeteria, students are expected to eat a limited selection of unimaginative foods day after day after day. Probably the most pernicious aspect of the National School Lunch Program isn't the myriad shortcomings of the food, but rather its uncanny knack for pushing even the brightest and most curious students into accepting, and then expecting, repetitive and uncreative meals.

By the time I finished high school, there were scarcely two dozen foods I regularly ate—and nearly all these foods were loaded with meat and dairy products. Jennifer was not going to let this happen to her son, and the daily lunches she fixes have made all the difference. Say words like "falafel," "roti," "penne," or "pad thai" to most seven-year-olds, and you'll be asked what language you're speaking. But to James, foods like these are all in a day's eating.

If you're a regular visitor to veganlunchbox.com, you know what it's like to continually wish you could reach into your computer display and pull out the day's featured meal. This book goes a step further, giving you the keys to James's lunchtime kingdom—complete recipes for dozens of his very favorite five-star meals. Make any one of these meals and you're bound to agree that these are all recipes worth going to school for.

Erik Marcus is the host of the Vegan.com podcast and the author of *Meat Market: Animals, Ethics, and Money.*

INTRODUCTION

I first became vegetarian at age fifteen after reading my mother's old, worn copy of the cookbook *Laurel's Kitchen*. I made the change for myself, for the earth, and for that "glossy black calf on its way to the slaughterhouse" that the book was so touchingly dedicated to.

After carefully studying their nutrition guidelines, I transformed myself from a teenager whose idea of a good lunch was a package of chocolate cupcakes and a jumbo cola (really), into someone who begged mom for special trips to the health food store. I tried my hand in the kitchen with mixed results (my first experience with tofu was less than stellar). I started baking 100 percent whole wheat bread—wrinkled, fragrant loaves that had the density and heft of wholegrain bricks.

But now that I was a vegetarian, I had to start packing my own lunch. Into my brown paper bag went a peanut butter and honey sandwich on inch-thick slices of extremely heavy whole wheat, an apple, and some carrot sticks. That was it—my lunch every afternoon for an entire school year.

Sure, it was a bit monotonous, even a bit grim at times. But I was determined that if this was what I had to do to save the animals, I would do it. I chewed away stoically on my sandwich, unaware of the world of bright and exciting vegetarian foods that awaited me in the future.

Over the years, I moved gradually from vegetarian to vegan. My love of the kitchen grew stronger and more passionate, and my cooking repertoire expanded considerably. Happily, my baking skills also improved (see page 220 for the bread that won me the coveted "Superintendent's Choice" award at our local county fair).

The summer my son turned seven and started preparing for first grade, I revisited the idea of packed lunches. I looked back on those peanut butter, carrot, and apple lunch bags, then down at my young son's head. There was no way he was going to put up with nothing but PB&J every afternoon for the next twelve years! There had to be more out there for vegan school kids.

I looked in every kid-friendly cookbook I could get my hands on. Some of the suggestions were great, but most of the "healthy" lunch ideas involved meat, cheese sticks, and hard-boiled eggs. That wasn't going to cut it for us.

Running out of inspiration there, I turned to the expert. "What do you want in your lunch on the first day of school?" I asked my son.

"Sushi!" he said.

I was both startled and thrilled. Sushi!?! How cool! It was light-years ahead of my own ideas.

From then on, I started keeping notes on various well-balanced lunch menus as they occurred to me. Soon I realized that not only did I have enough ideas to keep his meals healthy, well-balanced, and fun, but perhaps other vegan parents (or anyone trying to pack interesting, healthy lunches for themselves and their families) would also benefit from exploring these possibilities with me.

Thus, *Vegan Lunch Box* was born!

This book is filled with menus, recipes, suggestions, and ideas I have put to the test over the course of my son's first school year and on my Vegan Lunch Box blog. It has been shaped by my successes and even more importantly by my mistakes and by the many friends, blog readers, and fellow parents who shared their ideas and lunchtime tales with me.

It is my hope that this book will inspire you to create fabulous, healthy, well-balanced meals for your children. These menus are the perfect place to start building your own repertoire of school lunches your kids love. Knowing that you have packed them a lunch filled with the best in nutrition and with foods that they really enjoy will give you peace of mind during those long hours while they are away from home.

All the foods you will find in this book are 100 percent vegan. That means they contain no animal products of any kind—no meat, no dairy, no fish, no eggs, and no honey. This makes every lunch suitable for vegans and vegetarians, and for those with food allergies to fish, shellfish, dairy, or eggs. Many of the recipes are also free of other common allergens, such as soy, wheat, gluten, peanuts, and tree nuts (see the Allergen-Free Index on page 265).

Finally, don't forget the grown-ups in your life, including you! These menus are perfect for any adult who must eat away from home each day. Most parents also work outside the home, and dining out each afternoon can be expensive. When packing your child's lunch, make another one for yourself. You'll be saving money and time while eating a wonderful meal and will share a special connection to your child during the workday, when you both pull out your amazing vegan lunch boxes.

Happy eating!

P.S. Don't forget to check out the archives at the Vegan Lunch Box blog (www.veganlunchbox.com) for even more lunch ideas. You'll find a picture of every lunch I packed for my son during his first year of school (including pictures for most of the menus listed here). Each lunch includes a description, commentary, and success rating, along with helpful suggestions, occasional recipes, cookbook recommendations, and comments from readers. Don't miss it!

How to Use This Book

This book is divided into two parts: part 1, "The Lunch Menus," and part 2, "The Recipes." Each lunch box menu has been designed to offer a complete, well-balanced meal. I've tried to incorporate each of the following into every menu:

- **Whole Grains.** These are an excellent source of healthy complex carbohydrates, the perfect energy to fuel our bodies and get us through the day. This category includes not only whole wheat but also oats, barley, spelt, brown rice, quinoa, and even popcorn!
- **Protein.** Good vegan sources of protein include beans and legumes, soy products such as tofu, tempeh, edamame, soymilk, and yogurt, meat analogues such as veggie burgers, deli slices, chicken-less nuggets, etc., nuts and seeds (also good sources of healthy fats); and wheat gluten (seitan). Of course, protein is present to some extent in almost every food we eat.
- **Fruit.** Fresh, canned, dried, or thawed frozen fruit provide a wealth of vitamins and antioxidants.

- **Vegetables.** Fresh, canned, or cooked frozen veggies are a great addition to every lunch box and every meal. Offer a rainbow of colors each day—red tomatoes, orange pumpkin, green broccoli, purple cabbage—to provide your family with an enormous variety of health-protecting vitamins, minerals, and antioxidants.
- **Calcium.** Fortified juices and nondairy milks, soy yogurt, calcium-set tofu, almonds, kale, collards, broccoli, quinoa, figs, blackstrap molasses, and beans are just some of the good vegan sources of calcium you'll find here.
- **Dessert!** What kid doesn't appreciate just a bit of something sweet or fun to complete the meal? Throughout the book, you'll find recipes for homemade treats interspersed with examples of packaged vegan goodies available in grocery and health food stores. For more on dessert, see "Sweets and Treats" (page 231).

When trying these menus, feel free to make substitutions using what your children will eat or what you have on hand. If your children won't eat sweet potatoes, for example, substitute another orange vegetable like baby carrots. If they don't like kiwi fruit, how about some organic strawberries instead? Talk it over with your children and find out what they will eat.

WHAT'S TO DRINK?

Regarding beverages, don't forget to include lots of the best thirst-quencher of all: water. Bottles of water can even be frozen and used as ice packs in the lunch box; by lunchtime, they will have thawed enough to drink. Calcium-fortified nondairy milks and juices are also good choices.

"MY, WHERE DID YOU GET THAT LOVELY LUNCH BOX?"

The lunch box you see in the pictures (insert) is the Laptop Lunch System from Obentec in Santa Cruz, California. We love it! This fun, bento-inspired lunch box comes with removable containers in different sizes and colors and features a space for a fork and spoon. One of the larger containers has a lid to hold wet foods like applesauce or soy yogurt, and the set also comes with a tiny lidded container for things like dressing and dip. The other containers simply go into the lunch box without lids and the cover of the lunch box acts as a lid to hold them in place. Usually this is enough, but if I'm packing something very small, like peas and corn, I will cover the inner container with plastic wrap or foil just to be safe.

The entire lunch box then slips into an insulated carrying case with room for a Beverage container and an ice pack.

The Laptop Lunch System is available at www.laptoplunches.com or by phone at (831) 457-0301.

Part One

THE LUNCH MENUS

QUICK AND EASY

Let's start with menus that are fast and simple! This chapter is a great place to go if you are just learning to cook or don't have much time in the morning. Suggestions are included for convenient, store-bought snacks that can be easily tossed into the lunch box. If pre-packaged isn't your thing, plan ahead to have individual serving-size bags of these cookies or muffins at the ready in your freezer.

QUICK AND EASY 1

Lunch Nibbles (see below)
Easy Potato Salad (page 96)
Grapes
Back-to-School Chocolate Chip Cookies (page 232)
Beverage: Fortified nondairy milk

If you've been in an elementary school or mainstream supermarket lately, chances are you know all about this popular prepackaged lunch: processed cheese and deli meat are cut into little circles and served up on a plastic tray with just enough crackers to make a perfectly matched set of little cracker sandwiches. It's a great marketing concept with a lot of kid appeal, but you know from looking at the ingredients that there is nothing in this little lunch that you want children putting in their mouths!

So stick it to the man and make your own healthy vegan version, **Lunch Nibbles**: Cut circular shapes out of vegan deli slices (bologna, turkey, ham, salami, and so on) and/or vegan cheese slices using cookie cutters. Pair them with some savory rice crackers (smoked almond rice crackers are especially nice). Your child will be assembling cracker sandwiches with the best of them!

FRUGAL MOMMA TIP

Save the scraps of deli slices and cheese left over after making Lunch Nibbles to dice and sprinkle on soup, salad, or noodles later.

QUICK AND EASY 2

Tortilla Roll-Ups (page 138)
Salsa for dipping
Jicama sticks
Apple slices
Beverage: Horchata (see below)

A Mexican-inspired menu with some fun foods that may be new to you:

Jicama (HE-kuh-muh) is a round, brown tuber that is available in the produce section. Peel off the outer skin and cut the sweet white

FITTING IN

Some vegan kids don't care what others at school think about their lunch. They enjoy their meal regardless of what everyone else is eating (in fact, if they're lifelong vegans and healthy eaters they may even feel grossed out by what the other kids are eating). They're confident in the knowledge that what they're doing is right, kind, nutritious, and delicious, no matter what others may say.

For the rest of us mere mortals, however, peer pressure can have a significant impact on what our kids want to eat at school. Some children want nothing more than to fit in, look just like everyone else, and call absolutely no attention to themselves. That's where "fake meats" and many of the simple menus in this "Quick and Easy" chapter will help. Are all your child's peers eating nothing but turkey sandwiches and yogurt, and she or he desperately wants to join them? No problem—that's what vegan turkey slices and soy yogurt were born to do.

Matching what your child is eating to what is being served in the school cafeteria is another idea. See if you can get a copy of the cafeteria calendar. Is the school lunchroom serving hot dogs every Wednesday? Try sending Pups in Blankets (see page 167) or a veggie dog in a bun that day. Spaghetti and meatballs every Friday? Turn to page 159 for a recipe for pasta with Lentil-Rice Balls, a dish that will fit in quite nicely. You get the idea.

But perhaps your kid is the kind who enjoys a bit of attention, especially if that attention is in the form of the envy of their peers. Who can help but feel jealous when they see these amazing, colorful, well-balanced, exciting lunches, so obviously made by hand with great love? Check out the fun gourmet and exotic lunch menus in following chapters for the student who gets a kick out of showing off his or her vegan stuff.

Whatever your child's style, it's important to respect it. Communicate with them about what they want and pack them lunches in their style. Lunchtime should be something that they look forward to, both for the food and for the free time with their friends. And speaking of friends, sending a batch of Back-to-School Chocolate Chip Cookies (page 232) or Triple Chocolate Cupcakes (page 253) for your child to share doesn't hurt, either!

flesh into slices or spears. Eaten raw, it tastes something like a cross between an apple and a potato. Look for smooth-skinned, small jicama; the smaller ones are usually the sweetest.

Horchata is a traditional Mexican beverage made from sweet cinnamon-flavored rice milk. Rice Dream has recently come out with an all-natural version that's available in aseptic containers in the nondairy section of natural food stores.

APPLE PACKIN' TIP

Place apple slices in a small bowl and cover them with orange juice or natural citrus soda. Let them soak briefly then lift the slices out and shake them off. Pack in an airtight container or plastic bag. The citrus will keep the apples from turning brown before lunchtime arrives!

QUICK AND EASY 3

Nut Butter and Jelly Cutouts (page 133)
A baby banana
Carrot and celery sticks
Easy Ranch Dip (page 106)
Beverage: Cultured soy smoothie

Put a fun new twist on good ol' PB&J with some cookie cutters! Add a mini banana and some veggie sticks with ranch dip, and you have a classic kid's lunch combination.

Baby bananas are becoming more widely available in American supermarkets and are a perfect fit for the lunch box. These pint-sized beauties are a natural banana variety that grows to about half the size of a regular banana. Look for them next to the regular bananas in the produce section. And here's an interesting tip: they peel best from the bottom.

Cultured soy smoothies (like Silk Live! and WholeSoy & Co.) are a sweet, easy way to boost your child's nutrition at lunchtime. They are fortified with calcium, rich in soy protein, and contain the live active cultures that make yogurt so good for your intestinal well-being.

PEANUT PACKIN' TIP

Check with your children's school before sending them in with anything containing peanuts or peanut butter—some children are deathly allergic. If your child can't take peanuts to school, try replacing peanut butter with other butters such as cashew, almond, sunflower seed, or soy nut.

QUICK AND EASY 4

Pups in Blankets (page 167)
Ketchup or mustard
Kiwi fruit
Cooked frozen vegetables
Two crème-filled sandwich cookies
Beverage: Fortified nondairy milk

A good choice for those days when your child's school cafeteria is featuring corn dogs. These soy pups are rolled and baked in a delicious blanket of dough—no pigs in here!

Cooked frozen vegetables like peas, carrots, and corn are a convenient way to add vegetables to your child's meals. Cook according to package directions, drain well, and pack in a sealed container. Don't worry about the temperature; most children adapt to eating cold veggies without complaint and may even prefer them (think of the cold peas and beans you find at salad bars).

On the side is a sweet **kiwi fruit**. Did you know that one kiwi fruit has over 100 percent of your vitamin C for the day? Peel off the fuzzy skin with a paring knife and cut it into wedges or slices, or try eating it a different way: Cut the kiwi in half without peeling and scoop out the flesh with a spoon.

A surprising number of **crème-filled sandwich cookies** are vegan. Even several varieties of Oreos are now vegan! Look for organic varieties like Newman's Own in the health food section of the supermarket. Always check the ingredients on the label to be sure.

QUICK AND EASY 5

Mini bagels with vegan cream cheese
Green Beans and Carrots in a Tarragon Vinaigrette (page 98)
Red grapes
Animal crackers or alphabet cookies

Another simple, satisfying lunch that's easy to throw together on a hurried morning. But even though it's fast, it's still filled with fresh fruit, fresh green and orange vegetables, and healthy fats and proteins from nuts, seeds, and soy.

Mini bagels, available in most supermarkets, are the perfect size for little hands and mouths and fit nicely in a lunch box container. Younger children with smaller appetites may find one mini bagel suits them well. Throw in two or three for those with a bigger appetite.

Vegan cream cheese is available in the refrigerated section of most health food stores and many supermarkets. Tofutti "Better

Than Cream Cheese" and WholeSoy are two common brands. Look for plain vegan cream cheese or flavors like chive, garlic, vegetable, or berry.

Several brands of **animal crackers** and **alphabet cookies** are vegan (always check the ingredients to make sure). Newman's Own Organic Chocolate Alphabet Cookies and Barbara's Bakery Snackimals are two to look for. If using alphabet cookies, sort through and find the letters of your child's name or some other special word for them to puzzle out at lunchtime.

QUICK AND EASY 6

Vegan Deli Slice Roll-Ups (page 139)
Corn Tires (see below)
Melon balls
Pumpkin Carob Chip Muffins (page 214)

Vegan Deli Slice Roll-Ups are a big hit in our household. They are filling, high in protein, and easy to eat with the fingers, making them ideal for kids with limited lunch time. Alongside the roll-ups, a whole-grain pumpkin muffin is both a treat and a clever way to sneak in a serving of orange vegetables and ground flaxseed.

Corn Tires are little circular slices of corn-on-the cob (thanks to Liam for teaching us their proper name). They make a fun finger food for the lunch box and are easy to prepare: cook frozen corn-on-the-cob according to package directions, then cut into "tires" with a very sharp, heavy kitchen knife. If using fresh corn, cut the slices first, then boil until tender.

Use a melon baller to scoop out balls of fresh watermelon, cantaloupe, or honeydew. The balls of fruit are fun to eat and visually appealing, especially when mixed with round grapes or fresh blueberries. Making the **melon balls** is fun, too; ask your son or daughter if they'd like to scoop while you get the rest of the lunch box ready to go.

QUICK AND EASY 7

Pita Sandwich with Flaxy Hummus (page 135) and
   Oven-Dried Tomatoes (page 200)
Cucumber spears
Lemon soy yogurt topped with frozen blueberries
Sharkies

Several brands of **soy yogurt** are available at most grocery and health food stores today. We like to top our yogurts, flavored or plain, with generous servings of frozen fruit; by lunchtime, the fruit will have thawed and can be stirred into the yogurt for extra flavor.

Sharkies are fish-shaped gummy snacks that are wheat-free, gluten-free, fat-free, vegan, and all-natural. They are available at R.E.I. and some health food stores and on the Web at www.vegan essentials.com.

TASTE BUD TIP

I find that most kids I meet have more sensitive taste buds than the adults I know. Many dishes that taste just right to my husband or me taste "too spicy" or "too sour" to our son. When you try out some of the recipes in this book, such as Easy Hummus (page 105), keep in mind that I have created them with young, sensitive palates in mind. If you know you like your dishes hot and spicy, feel free to bump up the amount of seasoning.

QUICK AND EASY 8

Veggie Burger (see below)
Sweet Potato Oven Fries (page 86) or raw sweet potato spears
Wheat-Free Apple Crisp (page 254)
Beverage: Amazake

Oven-roasted sweet potato spears are simple to make and deliciously addictive. But if your child does not like cooked sweet potatoes (or you don't have the time to roast them on a given morning), try serving peeled, thinly sliced **raw sweet potato spears** instead; they have a sweet crunch like carrot sticks.

Amazake is a naturally sweet cultured rice drink available in a wide variety of flavors at natural food stores. It has a creamy, smoothielike consistency. Our favorite flavors are hazelnut and almond.

There are dozens of vegan **veggie burgers** on the market today. You can find them in the freezer, refrigerator, or even the canned food section of almost any grocery or health food store. We especially like the dried veggie burger mixes that you add water to and form into patties; these economical dried mixes can sometimes be found sold in bulk bins, saving money and packaging. Some veggie burgers taste quite a bit like meat; others taste more of brown rice, beans, mushrooms, or mixed veggies. Try them all and find out which ones you prefer.

Prepare the burger patty by frying it in a nonstick skillet with a drizzle of olive oil or according to package directions. Top with a slice of vegan cheese, if desired. Cover the pan to retain heat and cook until the cheese is warmed through.

Meanwhile, heat a large nonstick or cast-iron skillet over medium heat. Add a drizzle of olive oil to the pan. Slice the bun in half and place cut-side down in the pan. Sear the bun until it is toasted and warmed through, about one minute. Pan-toasting the bun adds a nice flavor and keeps the bread from getting soggy in the lunch box.

Spread the bread with Vegenaise and/or ketchup and mustard if desired. Place the burger patty inside the bun topped with your assortment of fresh veggies (if you won't be eating the burger for a while, you may wish to pack the vegetables separately in a resealable plastic bag, then add them at mealtime). Wrap the sandwich in parchment paper and/or foil and pack in a sealed container.

QUICK AND EASY 9

Beans and Dogs (page 145)
Baked pita chips
Cucumber crescents and edamame
Chocolate Banana Pudding (page 248) or a nondairy
    vegan pudding cup

Nothing could be simpler than serving up some warm baked beans mixed with veggie hot dog bites. It's always a real kid pleaser!

Baked pita or **bagel chips** are a great alternative to regular deep-fried potato chips. Look for low-salt varieties for all the crunch without all the sodium.

Toss together some peeled, seeded **cucumber crescents** (cut cucumber in half the long way and use a melon baller to scoop out the seeds, then slice into thin crescents) and shelled edamame (see page 69) for a new, tasty veggie combination.

If you don't have time to make this tasty homemade pudding ahead of time, pick up some **nondairy vegan pudding cups** at the store. Several varieties of pudding made from soy or rice milk are available. Look for it in the refrigerated section at your health food or grocery store.

QUICK AND EASY 10

Grilled Pepperoni Sandwich (page 130)
Sneaky Momma's Tomato Sauce (page 109) or store-bought
   pizza sauce
Broccoli Piccata (page 192)
A nectarine
A piece of vegan candy

Here's a quick lunch that's filled with flavor. A pepperoni-mozzarella sandwich tastes just right dipped in tomato or pizza sauce; lightly steamed broccoli shines when topped with vibrant lemon, garlic, and caper sauce. Throw in a sweet nectarine and a vegan candy treat and you've got yourself a lunch!

There are numerous **vegan candies** on the market, so there's no need to despair come lunch or holiday time. Dozens of mainstream kid favorites like AirHeads, Pez, Jujyfruits, Twizzlers, and SweeTarts are free of animal products. My personal favorite is the Mary Jane—old-fashioned peanut butter and molasses taffy, with what I think are the cutest candy wrappers ever (if I ever learn to decoupage, I'll be making something with Mary Jane wrappers).

For a list of more vegan candies and snacks, as well as some of the animal ingredients to watch out for, visit www.petakids.com/candy.html.

QUICK AND EASY 11

Chickpea Salad (page 94) in a whole wheat pita pocket
Green grapes and fresh mandarin orange slices
Jicama and carrot sticks, sugar snap peas, and red cabbage
   slices with Easy Ranch Dip (page 106)
Beverage: Vegan Hot Cocoa (see below)

We were all quite impressed by the rich flavor of this "chickeny" chickpea salad when I first made it—so impressed, in fact, that we made another batch for lunch the very next day! Try it in a pita pocket or on a bed of mixed greens.

Red cabbage makes a tasty addition to a selection of veggie sticks. Slice the cabbage into finger food–size strips. Pack them with celery, jicama sticks, sugar snap peas, and/or baby carrots. Include a container of Easy Ranch Dip (page 106) or any favorite salad dressing for dipping.

Vegan Hot Cocoa packed in an insulated container can feel nourishing and cozy on a chilly school day, and it's a cinch to make: For every 1 cup of fortified nondairy milk, whisk in 1 heaping teaspoon of cocoa powder or roasted carob powder and 2 heaping teaspoons of sugar. Heat in a saucepan or microwave, stirring or whisking frequently, until hot. Pack the cocoa in a preheated insulated food jar or beverage flask. Don't forget to include a straw, cut to fit into your lunch box if necessary.

QUICK AND EASY 12

Layered Bean Dip (page 107)
Baked Tortilla Chips (page 65)
Red, yellow, and orange bell pepper strips
Fresh papaya
Maple sugar candy
Beverage: Fortified nondairy milk

Refried beans and corn chips are an easy lunchtime snack, but that doesn't mean they have to be boring. Use the simple recipe on page 107 to turn plain refried beans into a zesty dip filled with layers of avocado and vegan sour cream. Serve with some bright bell pepper strips in shades of red, orange, and yellow for even more color and zip.

When packing chunks of fresh, luscious **papaya**, add a squeeze of lime juice. It will keep the papaya fresh and add a lovely brightness to the fruit's flavor.

Some vegans don't eat white sugar because of concerns about the use of animal bone char in the production of some cane sugar. If you wish to avoid white sugar but still have a sugary melt-in-your mouth treat every now and again, **maple sugar candy**—candies made entirely from maple syrup that has been crystallized and set in a decorative mold—can be a sweet alternative. Look for maple sugar candy in health food stores and gourmet markets, especially around the winter holidays.

RISE AND SHINE

Here are some lunches made for us morning people! Getting up a little early can make the difference between a boring same-old lunch and a fantastic culinary adventure. But don't worry! Most of these dishes can still be made ahead, just in case you'd rather sleep in.

RISE AND SHINE 1

"Eat Your Oatmeal" Pancakes (page 156) with
    maple syrup
Vegan breakfast sausage
Almond Buttered Sweet Potatoes (page 190)
Fresh organic strawberries
Beverage: Calcium-fortified orange juice

Pack up a "brunch-for-lunch" for a fun new twist on lunchtime. The next time you make pancakes for breakfast, cook a few extra "silver dollar"–size pancakes for the lunch box. Pack them cold along with a tiny container of syrup for dipping. Use your favorite vegan pancake recipe, or try our wheat-free favorite (page 156).

Vegan breakfast sausage is available in preformed links or patties or in unformed rolls that you can shape into patties or fry in crumbles. Look in the freezer and refrigerator sections at your supermarket. Prepare the sausage according to package directions.

Did you know that the calcium in most **calcium-fortified orange juice** (calcium citrate) is actually more bioavailable than the calcium in cow's milk? (Source: *Raising Vegetarian Children* by Joanne Stepaniak and Vesanto Melina.) What a simple way to boost calcium intake during the day!

RISE AND SHINE 2

Cream Cheese Spirals (page 68) and Tapenade Spirals (page 69)
Fruit salad
A vegan snack bar
Beverage: Vegetable–fruit juice blend

Fruit salad is a great way to keep fruit fun and increase the variety of fresh fruits in your day. Toss together slices of apple, orange, and banana and add some washed fresh berries or canned pineapple chunks or use a mixture of whatever fresh fruits you have available.

Healthy, vegan-friendly **snack bars** are proliferating like mad in the marketplace! For example, dozens of traditional granola bars made from oats, sweeteners, dried fruits, or vegan chocolate chips are available (watch out for added dairy or honey), as well as many "sports bars" with added protein powder and vitamins. We love the new lines of snack bars, like Larabar and Clif Nectar bars, made from dried fruits and nuts. They contain no added sweeteners, wheat, gluten, or soy and are made with a minimum of ingredients and processing. They taste great!

Vegetable–fruit juice blends are an interesting way to get your kids to "drink their vegetables." Look for brands that are heavy on the fruits and veggies, light on the high-fructose corn syrup.

RISE AND SHINE 3

Easy Pasta and Beans (page 154)
Seedless watermelon
Baby carrots
Nut and Seed Butter Cookies (page 242)
Beverage: Fortified nondairy milk

This is one lunch my son would be happy to eat every day! Most kids I know love pasta in all its forms, and this flexible recipe allows you to mix-and-match. It's a quick and simple recipe to fall back on in a pinch. If you use different pasta shapes and beans each time, it will always feel fresh and new.

RISE AND SHINE 4

Sausage biscuits (vegan sausage with
   Spelt Biscuits (page 216)
Perfect Hash Browns (page 201)
Ketchup
Vanilla soy yogurt topped with frozen mixed berries
Greg's Granola (page 71)
Beverage: Calcium-fortified orange juice

Here's a hearty, satisfying lunch, reminiscent of the breakfasts at certain fast food chains. Start with one or two **sausage biscuits**: prepare store-bought vegan breakfast sausage patties according to package instructions. Sandwich each patty inside a fresh-baked Spelt Biscuit (page 216) and add a layer of Vegenaise and/or ketchup if desired. A slice of vegan cheese is also an option.

Some crispy hash browns are a perfect side dish, packed with a small container of ketchup.

For a calcium-rich dessert, top vanilla soy yogurt with frozen fruit that will be thawed and ready to eat by lunchtime. Include a tiny container of homemade granola on the side to sprinkle on top for a healthy yogurt "parfait."

ORANGE ALERT

Carrots and other orange vegetables—such as sweet potatoes, pumpkin, and winter squash—are excellent sources of alpha- and beta-carotene. Try to include a serving of orange vegetables in your family's diet each day. Coconut Carrot Rice Pudding (page 152) is a delectable place to start.

RISE AND SHINE 5

Coconut Carrot Rice Pudding (page 152)
Blackstrap Gingerbread (page 207) with
    Lemon Sauce (page 208)
Applesauce cup
Soy jerky

This may seem like a lunch full of desserts, but there is a lot of nutrition hidden in these irresistible dishes! The slightly sweet Indian-inspired rice dish is filled with whole-grain brown rice, carrots, and heart-healthy fats from flaxseed and pistachios. The blackstrap molasses in the gingerbread is a great vegan source of iron and calcium, and the applesauce provides fiber, vitamin C, and potassium.

Soy jerky is one of my son's favorite treats. Chewy jerky is a portable, protein-rich food to snack on at lunchtime, when hiking and camping, or on road trips. Several brands are on the market now, with flavors ranging from gentle to superspicy.

RISE AND SHINE 6

Sweet Cornbread (page 217)
Linda's Collard Greens (page 199)
Fruit leather
Beverage: Fortified nondairy milk

For those of you not familiar with **black-eyed peas**, these little white field peas with black spots have been a dietary staple in the American South for over three hundred years. Available dried, canned, or in the freezer section, black-eyed peas are traditionally eaten for good luck on New Year's Day. They have a pleasant, mild flavor and are an excellent source of calcium, folate, and vitamin A.

If you have a bag of frozen black-eyed peas, you can whip up some **Black-Eyed Peas and Carrots** in a flash:

Empty a 16-ounce bag of frozen black-eyes into 4 cups boiling water and simmer for 10 minutes. Add 1 cup of chopped carrots, 1 minced garlic clove, and herbs and spices to taste (I like to add a generous pinch of oregano, thyme, and paprika). Simmer for another 5 minutes or so, until the carrots are barely tender.

Pack your pretty black eyes in a preheated insulated food jar, alongside a mini loaf of Sweet Cornbread (page 217).

RISE AND SHINE 7

Tofu Fish Sticks (page 182)
Tater Tots
Cocktail sauce or ketchup
Lightly steamed broccoli florets
Grapefruit segments

These Tofu Fish Sticks have been one of the most requested recipes on the Vegan Lunch Box blog—everyone's crazy for these cute little fishies! They stay crispy and crunchy in the lunchbox.

Tater Tots are their perfect lunchtime partner. These miniature frozen hash browns are called "potato pom-poms" in Australia and the United Kingdom—how cute is that? Look for organic varieties in the freezer section of your health food store. Prepare according to package directions, and pack them covered with foil. Serve the fish and tots with a small container of ketchup or cocktail sauce so you can take them for a dip.

RISE AND SHINE 8

Quinoa Amaranth Timbales (page 169)
Slow Cooker Black Beans (page 204)
Steamed Swiss chard (see below)
Tangerine slices
Beverage: Horchata (page 6)

Timbales are savory custards shaped in molds. Not only is a dish of quinoa and amaranth ideally suited to making timbales, the grains are also highly nutritious. These two tiny grains are good sources of high-quality protein and minerals, including iron and calcium. They are also gluten-free, which is good news for those with gluten sensitivities.

Steamed Swiss chard is an easy, nutritious side dish: trim off the tough lower stems and wash one bunch of fresh chard leaves. Chop leaves and tender upper stems into small pieces, then steam over boiling water until tender, about 4 minutes. Pack and eat them cold with a sprinkle of balsamic vinegar, or mix them in with the warm Slow Cooker Black Beans (page 204).

RISE AND SHINE 9

Polenta Fries (page 84)
Barbecue sauce or ketchup
Toasted soy nuts (see below)
Raw cauliflower florets
Beverage: Calcium Smoothie (page 257)

Creamy, cooked polenta transforms into luscious Polenta Fries when chilled, sliced, and broiled. This easy recipe produces fries that are crisp on the outside and tender on the inside, without the splattering, spitting hot oil that frying polenta on the stove involves. They are perfect for dipping into your ketchup or—even better—your favorite barbecue sauce.

Toasted soy nuts are made by baking dried, soaked soy beans until they turn crisp and brown. They make a good high-protein snack to pack along in lunches, purses, or backpacks. A bit crunchier than peanuts, soy nuts are available in a wide variety of flavors, from hickory smoked to lightly salted. Soy nuts are also easy to make at home:

Cover dry organic soy beans with water and soak them overnight. Drain and spread the soy beans in a single layer on a cookie sheet. Roast at 350°F, shaking the pan once or twice, until the beans are well browned and crunchy, about 1 hour. While still hot, sprinkle the nuts with some soy sauce or Bragg Liquid Aminos and a few drops of liquid smoke flavoring and toss well. Store the soy nuts in an airtight container.

RISE AND SHINE 10

Tennessee Corn Pone Muffins (page 218)
Vegan Ham Cutouts (see below)
Linda's Collard Greens (page 199)
Fresh or canned peaches

Here's a lunch menu inspired by my favorite American regional cuisine: southern cooking! Corn and bean muffins and southern collard greens go nicely with **Vegan Ham Cutouts**: set out a collection of cookie cutters and let the kids punch fun shapes out of vegan deli ham slices. Save the scraps to use in soups and salads.

The state of Georgia is famous for its sweet, juicy peaches, so some sliced peaches, fresh or canned in juice, are a delicious dessert in keeping with the southern theme.

RISE AND SHINE 11

Play Pretzels (page 83)
Nut butter
Celery sticks
Cheesy Roasted Chickpeas (page 194)
Sliced star fruit and kiwi fruit
Beverage: Fortified chocolate soy or rice milk

Here's a lunch menu for those mornings when your child and you feel like spending some time in the kitchen together before heading off to school and work. Talk about your upcoming day as you take turns pinching off bits of dough to roll into creative and interesting shapes to make Play Pretzels. Shape the dough into hearts, spirals, snakes, numbers, and letters. Best of all, these little pretzels will taste great at lunchtime and remind your child of the fun he or she had with you.

Pack them with some celery sticks and a small container of your favorite nut butter for dipping. Add some crisp and chewy roasted chickpeas for protein and an unusual fruit to add even more fun shapes to the lunch box.

The **star fruit**, also known as Carambola, is a golden yellow, deeply ribbed tropical fruit with a mild, slightly sweet, slightly sour taste. Slice star fruit across the middle of the fruit to create five-pointed stars. Add the stars to a mixed fruit salad or sandwich them between circles of kiwi fruit for a fun effect.

RISE AND SHINE 12

Lunch Box Fondue (page 72)
Assorted fondue dippers (page 73)
Apple chunks
A square of sweet dark chocolate

Kids love to dip things! A Thermos filled with piping-hot vegan fondue turns vegetable eating into a party. Serve it with a wide variety

---

FANCY FORKWORK

Keep your eye out at thrift stores and sales for those little chocolate fondue sets; you may score a miniature fondue fork that fits nicely in your lunch box. Don't send one with a child to school, though—they're too sharp and pointy. Save the fancy fork for yourself and let the kids use a regular fork for dipping.

---

of the veggies your kids love—and maybe one or two they aren't sure about yet!

Apples also taste great dipped in a cheesy sauce, making them the perfect fruit for this meal. And a bit of sweet, dark chocolate for dessert doesn't hurt, either!

RISE AND SHINE 13

Vegan "chicken" nuggets (see below)
Baked potato chips
Raw veggie shapes
Cherry Chip Brownies (page 236)
Beverage: Fortified nondairy milk

Vegan chicken nuggets are a great finger food for lunchtime. Because they look and taste so much like the real thing, it's a nice "undercover vegan" lunch if your child is feeling sensitive. Several varieties are available now in the freezer section of health food and grocery stores. Look carefully at the label before buying your nuggets; many contain egg.

NO NUKES!

When making vegan chicken nuggets and patties, be sure to bake them in the oven instead of microwaving them. When microwaved, they tend to toughen and become too chewy when they cool. Follow the cooking temperature and time on the package.

READY AND WAITING

Let's hear it for lunches made the night before, ready and waiting for you when you wake up in the morning! Doing most of the work in the evening means a quick lunch box assembly the next day.

READY AND WAITING 1

Wheat Gluten Pot Roast and Gravy (page 184)
Potato "Beetles" (page 202)
Blanched green beans
Fruit gel cup
Beverage: Fortified rice or oat milk

Gelatin molds, squares, and snack cups are certainly a mainstay of the kid-food world. But when I discovered that gelatin is made from the boiled bones, skins, and tendons of animals, those sweet, jiggly desserts went off my list for good.

Now, there's good news: several companies are making vegan **fruit gel cups** that use carrageenan seaweed and locust bean gum instead of animal gelatin. Many brands and varieties are available, including some that are organic and all-natural. Look for prepared fruit and gel cups on the shelf in the canned fruit aisle at the supermarket or in the refrigerated section at your local health food store.

READY AND WAITING 2

Roasted Tomato Basil Soup (page 121)
Crackers with slices of vegan cheese
Trail mix (see below)
Cashew Crispy Squares (page 234)

Warm, comforting tomato soup is the perfect lunch for a chilly autumn afternoon. Pack the soup along with some whole-grain crackers and slices of vegan cheese (see page 131). For a pretty lunch box presentation, use decorative cookie cutters to cut the vegan cheese slices into circles or square shapes that fit perfectly on top of your crackers.

It's easy to create your own one-of-a-kind, custom-designed **trail mix**: Set out jars or bowls of dried fruit, roasted or raw unsalted nuts and seeds, nondairy carob or chocolate chips, cereal, mini pretzels, and so on and let your children fill small containers or bags with their favorites. Some of our favorite combinations include pistachios with dried apricots and cherries; cashews with chocolate chips and raisins; almonds with dates and carob chips; and peanuts with dried pineapple and mini pretzels.

READY AND WAITING 3

Sneaky Momma's Black Bean Soup (page 124)
Baked tortilla chips
Applesauce with walnuts and Sneaky Cinnamon-Sugar
    (see below)

Get double-sneaky today with two stealth health foods! First, make a warm, creamy soup filled with undercover vegetables, hearty enough to satisfy even the hungriest tummy. Add some crunchy baked tortilla chips on the side.

Second, serve up a generous portion of organic, unsweetened applesauce with two omega–3-rich toppings packed separately to stir in at lunchtime.

Walnuts are the nuts highest in heart-healthy omega–3 fatty acids. I always keep a bowl of walnuts handy to crack open and snack on. Shell a handful just before packing and their flavor will be at its best. If you prefer your walnuts toasted, spread them on a baking sheet and toast for about 5 minutes at 350°F.

And here's a trick you might find yourself using often if your children are reluctant to eat their daily serving of ground flax-seed. It's **Sneaky Cinnamon-Sugar**: Stir together fresh, finely ground flaxseed with some natural dark brown sugar and a shake of cinnamon and store in a tiny lidded container. It tastes great on applesauce or hot breakfast cereal. Grind and mix only what you need for the day, as flaxseed is at its finest only when it's fresh.

READY AND WAITING 4

Creamy Cauliflower Soup (page 114)
Perfect Pepitas (page 82)
Blue Ribbon Bread rolls (page 220)
An orange
Two gingersnaps

This Creamy Cauliflower Soup is simple to make, but full of flavor and looks positively gourmet with its fancy green sprinkle of smoky, toasted **pepitas** (pumpkin seeds).

Vibrant **oranges** are a sweet treat rich in vitamin C and anti-oxidants. They can be packed in several different ways: peeled and divided into segments, cut into wedges, circles, or bite-size pieces, or left whole. If packing a whole, unpeeled orange, use a paring knife to cut away the top and bottom peel, then use a citrus peeler to score lines down the sides of the orange before packing. This makes for much easier peeling at lunchtime.

Gingersnaps are, you guessed it, yet another easy-to-find, usually vegan treat. Check the ingredients to be sure. Our favorites are the imported Swedish gingersnaps we find at gourmet import stores. Look for organic varieties sold at health food stores.

READY AND WAITING 5

Broccoli Fennel Soup (page 113)
Black sesame rice crackers
Tangerine slices
Fruit and Nut Bars (page 237)
Beverage: Soy smoothie

This soup has been one of our favorites for years. Broccoli and fennel are such a pleasing combination; the flavor of fennel fronds and ground fennel seeds brightens the earthy broccoli. Fennel, with its lovely mild licorice taste, is also thought to aid in digestion.

Snappy, gluten-free **rice crackers** are available in a wide variety of flavors. We found savory "black sesame" brown rice crackers seasoned with a touch of soy sauce paired beautifully with this soup, but unsalted sesame brown rice crackers are also a good choice.

Fortified **soy smoothies** might be a good option if your growing student is looking for some extra calories and protein. Smoothies are available in cans, bottles, and aseptic packages. They usually contain fruit and fruit juice mixed with soymilk and soy protein powder.

Try to find smoothies that are heavy on the fruit and soy and light on the high-fructose corn syrup and sweetener. You can also make your own by adding some flavored protein powder mix to regular soymilk and/or fruit juice.

READY AND WAITING 6

Peanut Butter and Jelly Muffins (page 213)
A frozen snack tube (see below)
Popcorn
Beverage: Vegetable juice

Here's a different twist on that old standby, PB&J: peanut butter muffins topped with chopped peanuts and filled with a pretty piping of fruit jam.

Snack tubes filled with sweetened yogurt are wildly popular today. What to do if your nondairy kids are pining away for squishy food-in-a-tube? Look for applesauce and applesauce/fruit blend snack tubes at your local grocery store, or make your own **homemade snack tubes**:

Fill a snack-sized resealable plastic bag with ½ cup soy yogurt or applesauce, or a mashed ripe banana mixed with mashed strawberries. Add extra goodies as desired (small pieces of dried or frozen fruit or small vegan chocolate or carob chips). Press the yogurt or fruit sauce into a tube-shape at the bottom of the bag. Squeeze any air out of the baggie and seal it shut, then freeze overnight. In the morning, cut a small slit in one corner of the bag before putting it in the lunch box. At lunchtime, your child can finish tearing off a small corner of the bag and squeeze the cool custardy treat into his or her mouth to eat.

A serving of fresh-popped **popcorn** packed in a resealable plastic bag also makes an easy, fun lunchtime snack. Don't forget to sprinkle it with the classic vegan popcorn topping: **nutritional yeast flakes**. We wouldn't dream of eating popcorn in our house without a sprinkling of our beloved "cheesy flakes."

But what is nutritional yeast? The tasty, bright yellow flakes are an inactive yeast grown especially for human consumption. Don't confuse them with the active dry yeast used to make bread, or with brewer's yeast, a bitter by-product of the brewing industry. Sprinkle them over popcorn, pasta, soups, or casseroles—anywhere you would sprinkle cheese or salt—for a great "cheesy" taste. Nutritional yeast is a rich source of protein and amino acids; look for "vegetarian support formula" for added Vitamin B_{12}. Nutritional yeast flakes are available in canisters or in bulk bins at the health food store.

MIGHTY MUFFINS!

Talking lunches with my vegan friend Martie and her teenage son inspired me to start thinking about the perfect lunch for a busy teen. It would have to be something lightweight, portable, quick to eat, and not too "strange." Muffins fit the bill perfectly! You can bake large batches of muffins on the weekend and freeze them in individual plastic bags. They'll be ready to toss into a backpack at a moment's notice. And once you've mastered the muffin, the creative ideas are endless! A tasty whole-grain muffin can contain vegetables (think zucchini, carrot, pumpkin), fruits (blueberries, banana, dried fruit), nuts and ground flaxseed for healthy fats, calcium-fortified soymilk, or even protein powder for the growing athlete.

READY AND WAITING 7

Full Meal Muffins (page 212)
Baby carrots
Easy Ranch Dip (page 106)
A Lady apple
Trail mix (page 28)
Beverage: Vegetable juice or fortified nondairy milk

The Lady apple is a tiny apple with a pretty red blush, available during the winter months. These apples are the perfect size for packing whole for those with smaller appetites.

READY AND WAITING 8

Veggie Tea Sandwiches (page 141)
Blueberry Lemon Mini Scones (page 209)
Fresh strawberries and purple grapes
Beverage: Kid's Iced Tea (page 258)

I just love traditional English High Tea—classical music in the background, little sandwiches with the crusts cut off, tiny scones and tarts, a sweetly scented cup of Earl Grey. Nothing could be more delightful on a spring afternoon.

In that spirit, here's an English tea service translated into a lunch box–friendly meal. An assortment of little sandwiches with their crusts cut off (how much more kid friendly does it get?) lined up beside two sweet mini scones and a colorful serving of fruit. Instead of hot tea, try this berry-flavored herbal iced tea with no caffeine, sweetened with apple juice ice cubes.

You can make the sandwiches and even the scones in the morning, but don't forget to start the tea and ice cubes the night before.

READY AND WAITING 9

Pizza Shop Breadsticks (page 227)
Sneaky Momma's Tomato Sauce for dipping (page 109)
Frozen vegetable and bean medley
Fresh blueberries and sliced fresh plums

These "cheesy" garlic breadsticks get their delicious taste from a mixture of sesame seeds and nutritional yeast. Enjoy them plain or dip them in a tangy tomato sauce.

Pick up some **frozen vegetable medleys** at the grocery store for quick veggies with no prep work; our favorite is a mixture of broccoli, carrots, and green, white, black, and kidney beans. Prepare them according to package directions and top with a spray of Bragg Liquid Aminos or low-sodium soy sauce.

READY AND WAITING 10

Hearty Chili Spuds (page 151)
Mixed green salad with Asian Miracle Dressing (page 92)
Banana-Pineapple Fruit Salad (see below)

This filling hot lunch is just right on a cold, rainy school day. A piping-hot serving of stick-to-your-ribs chili waits to be spooned over a hearty baked potato.

This **Banana-Pineapple Fruit Salad** has been a big favorite with the kids in our family for generations:

Combine equal parts fresh pineapple and banana slices and drizzle with a bit of agave nectar or Suzanne's Just-Like-Honey (page 241). Top with lightly toasted walnuts. The acidic pineapple and drizzle of "honey" keeps the bananas from getting too brown before lunchtime.

READY AND WAITING 11

Mini Wellingtons (page 76)
Peas and carrots
A sliced pear
Sugar wafer cookies
Beverage: Fortified nondairy milk

Sometimes visitors to the Vegan Lunch Box blog leave comments on which lunch is their favorite. I have to say, this one is mine! Beef Wellington is a traditional English dish made from a fillet of beef wrapped in pastry and baked. This vegan version is a savory mini loaf of nuts, rice, and beans wrapped in a puff pastry crust. The crispy, flaky puff pastry makes this dish supremely decadent and incredible to look at, and the inside loaf is rich, savory, and satisfying.

Keep an eye out for vegan **sugar wafer cookies**—light, airy wafer squares filled with creamy fillings. Some common brands include vegan flavors (check the ingredients to make sure). Match the criss-cross design of your wafer cookies to the criss-cross you make on your Wellington, and you'll be oh-so-coordinated!

READY AND WAITING 12

Mini Vegan Pizzas (page 160)
Spinach-pear salad with Raspberry Vinaigrette
    (see below)
Beverage: A can of natural, fruit-sweetened spritzer
    or soda

Who doesn't love pizza? Choose from four fantastic vegan pizza toppings and bake a pizza custom-sized to fit in your lunch box.

For a different twist on the usual tossed green salad, add some chopped fresh or dried fruit to your favorite greens. For example, we like a combination of shredded baby spinach and chopped crisp winter pears, topped with almond slices, dried cranberries, and this sweet **Raspberry Vinaigrette**:

⅛ cup balsamic vinegar
⅛ cup seedless raspberry jam
¼ teaspoon Dijon mustard
A dash of toasted sesame oil
¼ cup walnut oil (or canola)
Salt and pepper

In a small bowl or liquid measuring cup, whisk together the balsamic vinegar, raspberry jam, Dijon mustard, and toasted sesame oil. Slowly drizzle in the walnut oil, whisking constantly. Season with salt and pepper to taste.

READY AND WAITING 13

Pasta with Sneaky Momma's Tomato Sauce (page 109)
Lentil-Rice Balls (page 159)
Pomegranate seeds
A square of sweet dark orange chocolate

Pasta of any shape can be tossed with a rich tomato sauce filled with veggies and fresh basil and kept warm in an insulated food jar until lunchtime. Pack Lentil-Rice Balls separately to keep them crisp, then mix them with the pasta at lunch.

Studies of **pomegranates**, those lovely ruby "jewels of winter," have lately brought to light their powerful health benefits. They are high in antioxidants—containing almost three times the total antioxidants of the same quantity of green tea or red wine. However, they can be quite messy to eat! At home I score the outside of the fruit, lay down some plastic sheeting, and let my little one rip into it and go to town. The mess becomes part of the fun!

If you'd like to prepare a pomegranate for neat lunchtime nibbling, carefully cut through the outer skin and pull the pomegranate apart with your hands. Remove the bitter, white inner membranes and gently pry the seeds out. They are tangy and sweet, perfect on their own or sprinkled on salad.

For dessert, Newman's Own Organics makes delicious **sweet dark orange chocolate**. Cut off a small piece for lunch rather than sending the whole bar.

READY AND WAITING 14

Broccoli Calzones (page 147)
Sneaky Momma's Tomato Sauce for dipping (page 109)
Fresh apricots
An Aplet or Cotlet

This lunch provides whole grains, protein, and a vegetable all in one neat Italian package you can eat with your hands. A little fruit and a special little treat complete the meal.

Aplets and Cotlets are jellied fruit candies made by a company here in the Pacific Northwest. These soft, chewy confections, rolled in powdered sugar, remind me of Turkish Delights. The company, Liberty Orchards, uses only plant-sourced pectin to make their Aplets and Cotlets—they contain no gelatin, eggs, or dairy products. To obtain these goodies for yourself, visit their website at www.aplets.com.

READY AND WAITING 15

Petite Pasta Salad (page 102)
Lightly blanched cauliflower and broccoli florets
Fastest Dip in the West (see below)
Fresh kiwi fruit and fuyu persimmon
Banana Oatmeal Cookies (page 233)

Most pasta salads feature big pasta shapes and tiny bits of vegetables. I turned the idea on its head for this recipe, which features great big chunks of healthy vegetables tossed with tiny nibbles of pasta.

Next to the pasta are lightly blanched cauliflower and carrots with what surely must be the **Fastest Dip in the West**: toss a spoonful of Vegenaise with a squeeze of fresh lemon juice, a pinch of pepper, and a pinch of dried dill weed.

LUNCH BOX NAPKINS

One morning, I carefully folded two cookies into James's paper napkin as a lunchtime surprise. The cookies came home still neatly wrapped and untouched. The real surprise was that James never used his napkin!

What can parents do to encourage kids to wipe their hands and face, even at school? Try this tip from the moms at veganlunchbox.com, and sew your own lunch box mini napkins! Use fun fabrics that your kids will enjoy; you can even reuse fabric from old tablecloths, shirts, and so on. The best part is that they can be washed and used over and over again, eliminating the daily waste of disposable napkins.

Creative mom Dee Ruff-Sloan was kind enough to share this easy pattern with us, and even made James some exciting "superhero" napkins that were the envy of his peers. Thanks, Dee!

100% cotton or cotton-poly blend fabric
Basic sewing supplies

Cut your fabric into a 12 x 6-inch rectangle. Fold in half with wrong sides together and press.

Set fabric $1/2$ inch from sewing foot and sew up the open edges, making sure to backstitch at the beginning and end. Clip stray threads. Use pinking shears on the rough edges of fabric.

Wrap your new napkin around some silverware (or some cookies) and tuck into your lunch box.

4

LUNCH BOX ADVENTURE

Sick of sandwiches? How about sushi rolls, Greek phyllo triangles, Ethiopian flatbread, or Cornish pasties instead? Look here to discover new foods from around the world. You won't believe how varied and exciting your vegan lunch box will be!

JAPANESE ADVENTURE 1

Edamame (page 69)
Sushi Rolls (page 178)
Soy sauce
Organic grapes
Botan Rice Candy

This is the lunch box that started it all—my son's very first packed lunch on his first day of elementary school! Of course, not all six- or seven-year-olds may be ready for sushi in their lunchbox, so give them a taste at home and see how they like it first. But be careful—you may find that you have a new sushi fiend on your hands!

Botan Rice Candy are chewy candies covered with edible rice paper that melts away on your tongue. They are available at most Asian grocery stores.

> ## BECOME A SUSHI ACTIVIST!
>
> After you know how to make sushi, consider volunteering to lead a sushi rolling party to raise money or awareness for animal advocacy. Of all the activities our local vegetarian group has organized, our summer sushi party is by far the most well attended. Everyone loves rolling and eating sushi, and omnivores are always amazed at the fantastic sushi we can create without using fish.

JAPANESE ADVENTURE 2

Inari Sushi (page 158)
Pickled ginger
Edamame (page 69)
Pear slices
Botan Rice Candy

Literally "fox sushi," **inari** is named after the traditional Japanese god of grain. *Inari* are sweet, seasoned pouches made from fried tofu and filled with delicious sushi rice.

This is a great sushi to start the kids out on if they're not sure about seaweed. As a child, I stuck to sweet-tasting inari for several years before graduating to nori rolls. Inari was a big hit at my son's kindergarten "World Feast" luncheon, where the kids cleared the sushi platter in record time!

JAPANESE ADVENTURE 3

Sunny Whole-Grain Sushi (page 176)
Ponzu Sauce (page 177) or soy sauce for dipping
Japanese Spinach (page 198)
Asian Salad with Orange Sesame Dressing (page 93)
Fresh mandarin orange slices and kiwi fruit

I've always been crazy for vegan sushi. But as you can see from the basic Sushi Rolls recipe (page 178), regular sushi uses white rice seasoned with a mixture of rice vinegar, salt, and lots of sugar. So although it's fun as an occasional treat, it's not something I want showing up in my lunch box every day. Happily, I've come up with a recipe for healthy, whole-grain sushi that lets me enjoy my tasty nori rolls without all that sugar and salt.

When preparing this sushi for your lunch box, include a container of regular soy sauce, low-sodium soy sauce, or Ponzu Sauce for dipping and a bit of wasabi if you like the heat.

JAPANESE ADVENTURE 4

Musubi (page 79)
Adzuki Beans with Pickled Ginger (page 189)
Japanese Spinach (page 198)
An Asian pear

It's back to Japan again for another Asian lunchtime favorite that may be new to you: musubi! Musubi (also called *onigiri*) are balls of Japanese sticky rice wrapped with nori seaweed and usually stuffed with an umeboshi plum. "You're the ume in my musubi" is a Japanese version of "you're the cream in my coffee."

Serve some flavorful Japanese adzuki beans with your musubi, along with some spinach and a crisp Asian pear for a complete, well-balanced Lunch Box Adventure.

GREEK ADVENTURE

Phyllo Triangles (page 164)
Fennel Cucumber Salad (page 97)
Gigantes Plakis (Greek "giant beans") (see below)
Paximadia Cookies (page 243)
Beverage: Organic grape juice

It's My Big Fat Greek Lunch Box! Here's a lunch menu celebrating the wonderful cooking of Greece.

First, golden phyllo triangles are filled with tofu, dill, and lemon, and baked. Kids will like how neatly they fit in their hands. Adults will like the same tasty triangles with added onions and spinach.

A clean, refreshing salad of fresh fennel dotted with capers and olives is a fitting side dish, along with **Gigantes Plakis**. These Greek "giant beans" are becoming easier to find in the deli case at gourmet food stores; look for them prepared in vinaigrette dressing. If you can't find Gigantes, regular deli three-bean salad would be a good substitute.

For dessert, try some crunchy twice-baked Paximadia Cookies with some refreshing grape juice. *Opa!*

ETHIOPIAN ADVENTURE

Split Pea Alecha (page 126)
Mixed Vegetable Wat (page 120)
Ethiopian Injera Bread (page 225)
Fresh casaba or honeydew melon

Here's a spectacular, luscious, Ethiopian-inspired lunch box. If you are lucky enough to live near an Ethiopian restaurant, you know that traditional Ethiopian cuisine is filled with mouthwatering vegetarian dishes made from lentils, split peas, vegetable stews, and cooked greens, seasoned with rich spices and hot pepper and served on top of injera, a flatbread made from nutritious teff flour.

James loves Ethiopian injera bread; he used to call it "silverware bread" because we eat Ethiopian food in the traditional manner, by scooping it up with torn-off pieces of injera—no silverware! Now he likes to top his injera with this stunningly green split pea alecha (stew) and call it "Martian Pizza."

ENGLISH ADVENTURE

> Cornish Pasties (page 153)
> Brazil nuts
> Fresh figs or fig bars
> Beverage: Fortified nondairy oat or multigrain milk

The **Cornish pasty** goes back hundreds of years. Miners in Cornwall, England, packed these savory hand pies filled with beef, potatoes, onions, and turnips to take into the mines. They made a nicely portable, handheld meal. Sometimes the pasties were filled with a bit of apple or jam at one end so you could eat through lunch and hit dessert! I wasn't that clever, though; these pasties are filled from end to end with savory diced potato, turnip, and vegan steak strips.

Did you know that **Brazil nuts** are actually seeds? The enormous Brazil nut tree produces hard pods resembling coconuts, containing ten to twenty-five seeds each. Very popular in the United Kingdom, Brazil nuts are eaten raw or roasted. They are an excellent source of protein, fiber, and selenium and are high in zinc, magnesium, and other minerals.

Figs are traditionally used dried in preserves, puddings, and cakes in England. But if you can find juicy green or brown fresh figs at the farmers' market or fruit aisle, they make a stunning fresh fruit for the lunch box. If you can't find fresh ones, there are a few vegan **fig bars** on the market; check the ingredients listed on the package to make sure. And by the way, did you know figs are a good source of calcium?

MEXICAN ADVENTURE

Spanish Empanadas (page 175)
Red Rice and Black Beans (page 170)
Mango, Jicama, and Cucumber Snack (see below)
Beverage: Lemonade

When I started the Vegan Lunch Box project, I had no idea how universal the hand pie was—portable, packable, handheld pies stuffed with savory fillings. Now I've made friends with the Italian calzone (page 147), Russian piroshki (page 168), Cornish pasty (page 153), and these Spanish empanadas! Any food wrapped in pie dough gets an immediate five-star rating in my household.

These easy empanadas are filled with spicy, taco-flavored veggie meat; include a small container of vegan sour cream for dipping. Also on the side, red rice looks vibrant sitting side-by-side with a serving of dark black beans.

Traditional **Mango, Jicama, and Cucumber Snack** tastes cool, light, and refreshing, just right next to the heavier empanada with rice and beans. I still remember when I bought my first paper cone filled with this intriguing fruit and vegetable combination from a street vendor at a Cinco de Mayo celebration.

Peel mango, jicama, and cucumber (or leave the cucumber peel on if it is organic) and cut them into long spears. Toss with a squeeze of fresh lime juice and sprinkle with salt and dried ground ancho chile or cayenne (optional).

MEXICAN ADVENTURE 2

Black Bean Tamales (page 146)
Salsa
Calabacita con Elote (page 193)
Fresh mango slices
Beverage: Horchata (page 6)

Delicious tamales—wedges of corn masa dough filled with luscious refried beans—served with salsa, Mexican zucchini, fresh mango, and sweet cinnamon rice milk make a fantastic lunch filled with the flavors of Mexico.

You could plan this for right after Christmas break, as tamale-making is a traditional holiday-time activity. Once you are comfortable making delicious tamales, quadruple (or more!) the recipe and invite some friends over for your own tamalada–a traditional tamale-making party. Your guests will be delighted when you send them home with their own package of gorgeous, handcrafted tamales.

INDIAN ADVENTURE

Aloo Samosas (page 143)
Massur Dal and Carrot Soup (page 118)
Cucumber Raita (page 95)
Fresh mango slices mixed with canned mandarin oranges

Here is a menu that hints at the wonders to be found in Indian cuisine. First, delicious little baked bundles filled with potatoes and peas, followed by a warm, satisfying soup made from red lentils and carrots, and finally a cool cucumber-yogurt salad. Fresh mango slices pair wonderfully with drained, canned mandarin orange segments for a sweet treat.

There is nothing I love more than Indian food. There was great happiness in our household the day we discovered an Indian restaurant opening just down the street from us. Unfortunately, my son finds many Indian dishes too spicy for his taste. So, for James and his wimpy-tongued Western compatriots, these simple Indian-inspired recipes hopefully have just enough spice to get them started on a fine lifelong addiction to Indian food, without sending them running for the tap.

VARIATION: Instead of yogurt salad and mango slices, try a mango-flavored cultured soy beverage or blend a handful of fresh or frozen mango with vanilla soy yogurt and ice or water. It tastes like the delicious mango lassi drinks served at Indian restaurants.

THAI ADVENTURE

Tofu Apple Spring Rolls (page 87)
Quick Peanut Sauce (page 108)
Ted's Asian Asparagus (page 205)
A fresh plum
Black Rice Pudding (page 247)

Here's a lunch box menu inspired by the flavors of Asia and the fresh fruits and vegetables of spring. Tender spring asparagus and a fresh plum or other springtime fruit go nicely with delicious rice paper wraps filled with tofu and crunchy cabbage.

At first glance, this may look like one of the more "grown-up" lunches in this book, and it certainly is sophisticated enough to impress the folks at the office. But give it a try with the kids, too—

chewy rice paper spring rolls filled with tofu and apples and dipped in peanut sauce can be a real kid pleaser, and a sweet pudding made with jet black rice is a delightful treat at any age!

THE WONDERS OF RICE PAPER

Rice paper wrappers are a fantastic alternative to bread for the gluten-intolerant. Look for them in packages at Asian markets. Dry and hard when purchased, they become soft and pliable with a quick soak in warm water. Wrap up any favorite salad or baked tofu to make a handy portable lunch.

FRENCH ADVENTURE

Ham and Cheese Croissant (page 222)
Haricot verts (see below)
Strawberries
Beverage: Hazelnut Soymilk (see below)

Here's a vegan culinary trip to France! There is nothing like the smell of hot, baking croissants wafting through the kitchen and the taste of one fresh from the oven. See if you can save any long enough to fill them with vegan ham and cheese for *un déjeuner délicieux* (a delicious lunch).

Classic French filet green beans or **haricot verts** are slimmer, smaller, and faster-cooking than regular Western green beans. The thin young beans have a delicate sweetness and great flavor. Look for them at farmers' markets and grocery stores. Blanch them briefly (4 to 5 minutes) in boiling salted water, until barely tender. Rinse the beans with cold water, drain, and pack.

Before I liked soymilk, I liked **Hazelnut Soymilk**: mix one cup of vanilla soymilk with one tablespoon of hazelnut syrup (the kind of bottled syrup used to flavor coffee drinks at espresso bars). The flavors are so right together—even soy haters may convert! Pack it cold with an ice cube or two or try warming it up and keeping it in an insulated beverage flask on a cold day. A soymilk "steamer" (hot, steamed milk with a bit of foam) flavored with a shot of hazelnut is my favorite drink to order at espresso stands that carry soymilk. Kids love it, too!

MONKEY MADNESS ADVENTURE

Tofu Lettuce Cups with Mango Chutney (page 89)
Hazelnut Banana Sandwich Bites (page 132)
Peas and carrots
Corn Tires (page 9)
Monkey Chow (fruit-shaped cereal)

Monkeys love to eat their fruits and vegetables! Pack your own little monkeys a fresh, fun mix of peas, carrots, corn, and Hazelnut Banana Sandwich Bites. A handful of Monkey Chow (dry, fruit-shaped breakfast cereal) makes a crunchy, fun dessert.

For more adventurous monkeys (and adults), these Tofu Lettuce Cups make a refreshing, satisfying lunch. Gingery tofu is paired with lively lime, coconut, and peanuts in a lettuce wrapper. Be sure to tuck in an ice pack or frozen water bottle to protect your lunch from the heat.

Enjoy your Monkey Madness Adventure, and then hit the local Jungle Gym for a little after-lunch swinging!

"MORE, PLEASE!"

Looking for more menu ideas and lunch box Adventures? Not to fear! Just visit the Vegan Lunch Box blog: veganlunchbox.blogspot.com.

Once there, you'll find dozens of creative ideas, pictures, and lunch box suggestions. Browse the entire blog archive month-by-month. You'll find an entire year of vegan lunches, including dishes from dozens of vegan and vegan-friendly cookbooks, all handily referenced and reviewed.

Many of the lunches feature ethnic menus like those in this chapter from around the world. In addition to all the menus you see here, you'll find Chinese, Australian, Jewish, Japanese, Indian, French dishes, and more, plus lots of good ol' American kids' cuisine—bologna and snack cakes, anyone?

SPECIAL OCCASIONS

Every day is a celebration, but special times call for extra-special lunches. Here are themed menus designed for those grand days—birthdays, holidays, graduation, and celebrations of the season. Let your little lunchers know how special they are by surprising them with these fun-filled holiday menus.

BIRTHDAY MENU

Your child's favorite lunch
Fluffy White Cupcakes or Triple Chocolate Cupcakes
  (pages 249 and 253)

Birthdays are the perfect time to bring a treat to share with the class or coworkers. Everyone, both young and old, veggie and omnivore, will love these incredible, decadent cupcakes. No one will ever guess that they contain no dairy or eggs!

We have a tradition in our family that the birthday person always chooses what we have for dinner. Why not extend this tradition to lunch as well? Let your child pick his or her favorite lunch menu, and don't forget to tuck a surprise birthday card into the lunch box!

SUGAR-FREE BIRTHDAY IDEAS

Who says sugar has to be part of every classroom celebration? If your family is trying to avoid the white stuff, try bringing a sugar-free treat to share instead. Fresh Fruit Kabobs (page 61) are colorful, fun, and easy. Nonfood items like pencils or little toys are another alternative.

FALL EQUINOX MENU

Savory Autumn Leaf Pies (page 172)
Pretzel sticks
Nut butter
Lima or butter beans
Apple slices

Leaves and sticks—it's what many people think vegans eat, isn't it? In celebration of the Fall Equinox, send your son or daughter to school with this earthy menu: savory **leaves** made from a barley poppy seed crust and filled with roasted autumn vegetables, alongside pretzel **sticks** with a small container of natural peanut or almond butter for dipping.

Throughout the school year as I posted lunch pictures on my blog at veganlunchbox.com, people asked me how I got my son to eat

lima beans. What was my secret recipe? It's simple: I open a can of lima beans, drain them, rinse them, and set them before him. It's one of his favorite beans, and he gets grumpy if he has to share. Look for canned limas at any supermarket; in some stores you can even find canned "chestnut" limas with beautiful brown speckling. Chestnut limas make an even lovelier, earthier-looking accompaniment to this fall feast.

MAKE IT SPOOKY!

Make this lunch extra-fun by decorating your lunch box with Halloween-themed stickers and toys. Last year, I used black cat stickers and Halloween-style spooky letters on the outside of the lunch box to warn the diner to "BEWARE" of what they would discover when the box was opened!

HALLOWEEN MENU

Scary Spider Sandwiches (page 136)
Gobblin' Fingers (page 70)
A pear
Beverage: Witches' Brew (page 259)

Here's a spine-tingling lunch for that spookiest of holidays, Halloween. "Spider" sandwiches creep around on a nest of "mummy wrappings," while Gobblin' Fingers await dipping. A murky bottle of Witches' Brew is sure to chill and delight.

THANKSGIVING MENU

Pumpkin Anadama Rolls (page 229)
Tofurky
Cranberry Sauce
Wild Rice Pilaf (page 187)
Native Blend Popcorn Balls (page 80)
Beverage: Concord grape juice

Here are some wonderful recipes that will give all the vegans in your life something to be thankful for at Thanksgiving dinner (not to mention making the animals thankful as well).

After your Thanksgiving feast, save some leftovers and put together this native foods–themed lunch box the next day. Sandwich a few slices of leftover **Tofurky** or other vegan roast in a Pumpkin Anadama Roll (page 229). Spread the sandwich with a bit of Vegenaise and/or cranberry sauce for a lovely post-Thanksgiving treat.

> ## ADOPT A TURKEY, DON'T EAT ONE!
>
> A picture of your family's own adopted turkey would be the perfect thing to tuck into this lunch box to give your loved one an afternoon smile. To adopt, visit www.adoptaturkey.org.

I like to use the time around Thanksgiving to highlight some of the foods that we eat that are native to North America. While your children help you pop popcorn or shape dinner rolls, tell them a little about the native foods that are featured in today's lunch:

- **Corn** was domesticated in central Mexico, then spread north, and was a major part of the Native American diet by Columbus's time.
- **Cranberries, blueberries,** and **concord grapes** are the top three Native American fruits that are commercially grown today.
- **Pecans** are the only major commercially grown tree nut that is native to North America. The name "pecan" is an Algonquin word, meaning a nut that must be cracked open.
- **Popcorn** was spreading through almost all the tribes of North and South America by the time the pilgrims arrived. To the early Native Americans, popcorn was a currency of trade and friendship and a symbol of hospitality.
- **Pumpkins** and squashes are also native to the New World. Native Americans grew pumpkins for food for thousands of years. Pumpkin was served at the first Thanksgiving and quickly became a staple in the diet of the first European settlers, as well.
- **Sunflower** was a common crop among Native American tribes throughout North America. Sunflower seeds were ground or pounded into flour, cracked and eaten, or even squeezed for oil.
- **Wild rice** is actually not rice but a native grass that grows in lakes and river beds primarily in areas west and north of the Great Lakes. The Algonquin, Ojibwa, Dakota, Winnebago, Sioux, Fox, and Chippewa tribes used wild rice as an important staple in their diets.

CHRISTMAS MENU 1

Best Brussels Sprouts (page 191)
Golden Chestnut Soup (page 117)
A clementine or satsuma
Gingerbread Vegans (page 238) with Gingerbread Vegan Icing (page 240)
Beverage: Soy nog

Here's a warm welcome to the wintertime holidays! Creamy, piping-hot Golden Chestnut Soup warms the tummy on a cold winter's day. Brussels sprouts have long accompanied chestnuts at holiday meals, and this meal is no exception; I find them addictive in this sweet, tangy sauce.

Clementines and **satsumas** are sweet, seedless mandarin oranges that become available each year around Christmastime. Pick some up for a special holiday treat and old-time stocking stuffer.

You can decorate your Gingerbread Vegans at home before you pack them, but they are really the most fun when you pack them naked along with some sprinkles and a miniature piping bag filled with icing, so the luncher can decorate the cookies right before eating them (see directions in the recipe).

And finally, what would the holidays be without some **soy nog**? I think Silk brand soy nog is one of the best things in life. Really, give it a try—it will nog your socks off!

CHRISTMAS MENU 2

Christmas Limas with Chestnuts and Brussels Sprouts
   (page 196)
A whole-grain dinner roll
Radishes, trimmed to look like peppermints
Fastest Dip in the West (page 38)
Star fruit and pomegranate seeds
Vegan Fudge (page 245)

Christmas lima beans pair beautifully with the traditional holiday mix of sweet chestnuts and brussels sprouts.

Radishes can be trimmed to look like peppermints: use a paring knife to scrape off strips of red skin to expose the white flesh. The effect is quite convincing; when I featured a picture of this lunch on my blog, many readers wrote to tell me they thought the radishes really were big Christmas candies!

VALENTINE'S DAY MENU

Tomato Roses on a Bed of Cannellini Been Puree
  (page 110)
Whole-grain crackers
Cherry Almond Mini Scones (page 210)
A piece of vegan dark chocolate

Send your sweethearts, big and small, out into the world this Valentine's Day with a special lunch that says "I love you!" First, roasted

---

VEGAN CHOCOLATE

Chocoholics, don't worry! Going vegan doesn't mean giving up your daily chocolate fix! Chocolate comes from a plant—the cacao plant—and is a vegan product in its natural state. Most chocolate is then combined with sugar and dairy to make the "milk chocolate" we find in most stores, but non-dairy chocolate is becoming more and more available.

Fantastic dairy-free dark chocolate can be found in most health food stores (but not all dark chocolate is dairy-free, so be sure to check the ingredients). You can also find an enormous selection of gourmet vegan chocolates online, including truffles, hearts, bunnies, and boxes of vegan cream-filled assortments. Check out sites like Vegan Essentials and Food Fight! Vegan Grocery (see Recommended Resources, page 261), or do a Web search for "vegan chocolate." You'll be amazed at the mouthwatering selection.

beets are shaped into hearts in a flavorful salad filled with fruits and vegetables. Then, parsley and tomato skins are used to create miniature red roses on a bed of rich cannellini beans.

For dessert, a sweet cherry and almond scone is a romantic rosy red. You could even shape your scones into hearts using large cookie cutters or a heart-shaped muffin pan. Follow the scone recipe on page 209, using the variation for Cherry Almond Mini Scones at the end.

Finally, don't forget to include a special Valentine's card or handwritten love note, along with that little bite of sweet dark chocolate for dessert (see page 59). Because what food says "love" like chocolate?

VALENTINE'S DAY MENU 2

Peanut Butter and Jelly Pop Hearts (see page 134)
An assortment of raw vegetables
Store-bought vegan salad dressing for dipping
Fresh strawberries
Beverage: Fortified nondairy milk

Here's a simpler, very kid-friendly Valentine's Day lunch menu, featuring an adorable heart-shaped pastry filled with nut butter and jam. Use a piping bag filled with icing to decorate the baked, cooled Pop Hearts with swirls and stripes or sweet sayings like "Be Mine" or "I Love You."

EASTER MENU

Sunflower Sandwich (page 137)
Honeybee No-Bakes (page 241)
Sprout Salad with Mandarin Orange Dressing
    (page 103)
A plastic egg filled with vegan jelly beans

This lunch box is a cheerful celebration of springtime! The sandwich is masquerading as a beautiful sunflower and has attracted a following of no-bake cookie bees that can't wait to take a taste.

The crispy sprout salad is a celebration of the new, emerging life of spring, especially when you take the time to grow the sprouts yourself. Don't forget to tuck in an ice pack with this lunch—sprouts will wilt quickly if they get warm.

Watch out when choosing **jelly beans**. Jelly beans and other jelly candies may contain gelatin and beeswax. For a list of vegan candies (including gelatin-free jelly beans) and other great Easter ideas, visit PETA's "Cruelty-Free Easter" page at www.peta.org/feat/easter/baskets.html.

GRADUATION PARTY!

Vegan Mini Pizzas (page 160) or Build-Your-Own-Tacos
  (see below)
Fruit Kabobs (see below)
Graduation Hats (page 251)
Beverage: Sparkling juices and seltzers

You've done it! You've survived another school year (and I'm talking to you parents and teachers as well as the kids)! Whether it's kindergarten, senior year, or somewhere in between, it's time to celebrate! Throw a graduation bash with an assortment of vegan pizzas or a **Build-Your-Own-Taco Buffet**: start with crisp corn taco shells and lay out a selection of taco toppers like taco-flavored veggie meat, refried beans, guacamole, vegan sour cream, black olives, shredded lettuce, tomatoes, and salsa.

Fruit Kabobs make regular fruit into something celebratory: alternate chunks of colorful fresh pineapple, grapes, strawberries, and tangerine segments on small bamboo skewers. If taking this to school or serving it to younger children, use small red coffee stir straws instead of wooden skewers for safety.

For dessert, bake a batch of chocolate cupcakes and use a bit of kitchen magic to transform them into Graduation Hats.

A LITTLE NOTE ON LITTLE NOTES

One afternoon in third grade, I opened my lunch bag and discovered a special note from my mom, jokingly referring to a funny story she had told me the day before. "Dear Jenna, Don't let a birdie poopoo on your head! Love, Mom!"

Now everyone knows that the mention of "poo" can send kids into fits of hysterics. I immediately shared this with the kids around me, and the giggling quickly reached a fever pitch. Suddenly, a large shadow loomed over us.

"Girls?" the teacher asked, "What's so funny? Ah. I'll take that, thank you."

I was mortified. Not only had I gotten us all in trouble, but my precious letter had been taken away from me. I never forgot that note from home, nor did I ever see it again.

Now, I've recovered enough from my childhood trauma to become a big fan of notes in the lunch box. I've built up a fun collection of little notes to tuck into lunches at random, including mazes, jokes, brain teasers, mini cards for holidays and special occasions, and sweet little illustrated notes that say things like "I'm Proud of You!"

Lunchtime notes can be a nice way to remind your children that even though they're away from home, you're still thinking about them. But please, nothing too hysterical, okay?

Part Two

THE RECIPES

APPETIZERS AND SNACKS

BAKED TORTILLA CHIPS

Buy baked, unsalted tortilla chips to cut out the fat and sodium of regular chips, or make your own from fresh corn tortillas.

About 2 tortillas
make a serving

Corn tortillas

Canola oil

Sea salt

Chili powder (optional)

▶ Preheat the oven to 350°F.

▶ Use a pizza wheel or sharp knife to cut the tortillas into strips or wedges. Brush both sides with canola oil and sprinkle with salt to taste and chili powder, if desired.

▶ Arrange the chips in a single layer on a baking sheet and bake until golden brown and crisp, about 15 minutes.

CHOCOLATE GRAHAM CRACKERS

These crisp, not-too-sweet crackers are just right eaten plain, spread with nut butter, or dipped into spicy pumpkin butter or apple butter. Homemade graham crackers are fun to make together. Let your young artists cut out the dough with cookie cutters and use a fork or toothpick to poke holes in the tops.

Graham flour is a coarse grind of whole wheat flour. If you can't find it at your local health food store, substitute regular whole wheat flour.

Makes about 3 dozen crackers, depending on the size you cut them

----

1 cup all-purpose flour

1 cup graham or whole wheat flour

1/4 cup sugar

1/4 cup cocoa powder (or carob powder)

1 teaspoon baking powder

1/2 teaspoon kosher salt

1/4 teaspoon cinnamon

1/2 cup nonhydrogenated margarine, chilled

2 tablespoons maple syrup

1/2 cup water

1 teaspoon vanilla

▸ In the bowl of a food processor fitted with the S blade, combine the flours, sugar, cocoa powder, baking powder, salt, and cinnamon. Pulse to combine. Dot the top of the flour mixture evenly with spoonfuls of the cold margarine. Process until the mixture resembles coarse meal.

▸ Add the maple syrup, water, and vanilla, and process until the mixture forms a dough.

▸ Scrape the dough out of the food processor onto a well-floured surface and form into a flat disk. Wrap the disk in plastic wrap and refrigerate for at least 1 hour.

▸ Preheat the oven to 350°F. Line two baking sheets with parchment paper and set aside.

▸ Working with half of the dough at a time and keeping the other half wrapped in plastic, roll the dough out on a lightly floured surface using a rolling pin. Roll to a thickness of about ⅛ inch (the thinner the crackers are, the crisper they will be). Cut out the crackers into squares, circles, or whatever shape you desire. Use a thin metal spatula to transfer the crackers to a baking sheet.

▸ With a fork, prick several holes in each cracker (this allows moisture to escape and makes the crackers crisp). Bake for 15 to 18 minutes, until the crackers are firm and lightly browned on the bottom. Don't worry if they are a bit soft; they will become crisper as they cool. Remove the crackers to a wire rack to cool completely before storing in an airtight container.

VARIATION: Sprinkle the tops with Perfect Cinnamon-Sugar (page 215) before baking.

WHY SHOULD SANTA HAVE ALL THE FUN?

On Halloween or All Souls' Eve (October 31), you can follow an old European tradition by leaving out a plate of circle-shaped Chocolate Graham Crackers as "soul cakes" for the wandering souls of the dead. The shape represents the circle of life and death.

CREAM CHEESE SPIRALS

These lovely cookie-size spirals filled with vegan cream cheese and fresh herbs or a zesty tapenade are the perfect addition to an appetizer or finger food tray and are fantastic in the lunch box.

Makes 20 spirals, about 4 servings

$^3/_4$ cup all-purpose flour

$^1/_4$ cup whole wheat flour

1 $^1/_2$ teaspoons baking powder

$^1/_2$ teaspoon kosher salt

4 tablespoons canola oil

4 tablespoons plain, nondairy milk, plus more as needed

6 tablespoons vegan cream cheese, room temperature

2 tablespoons minced fresh herbs (basil, parsley, dill, and thyme)

Freshly ground black pepper

▸ Preheat oven to 350°F. Line a baking sheet with parchment paper and set aside.

▸ Whisk together the flours, baking powder, and salt, then stir in the oil and milk to form a stiff dough (add a bit more milk if needed to hold the dough together). Turn the dough out onto a lightly floured surface and roll out with a rolling pin into an 8 x 11-inch rectangle. Spread on a thin layer of cream cheese and sprinkle with herbs and black pepper to taste. Starting at a long edge, roll the dough into a log, pressing firmly so that no pockets of air are trapped inside. Cut the dough log into twenty $^1/_2$-inch disks. Place on the baking sheet and bake until set and golden brown on the bottom, about 20 minutes.

VARIATION: Tapenade Spirals: follow directions above, substituting 4 tablespoons store-bought roasted red pepper or black olive tapenade for the vegan cream cheese.

EDAMAME

Edamame (eh-dah-MAH-may) are green baby soybeans, available in the freezer section of most grocery and health food stores. They are easy to prepare and fun for kids to eat; pick up a pod and pinch the soybeans out into your mouth.

You can also buy frozen edamame that are already shelled. These take up less space in the lunch box and are faster to eat (but not as much fun!). Prepare them as described above, or follow package directions.

Makes 3 to 4 servings	5 cups water, lightly salted 1 (12-ounce) package frozen edamame pods Garlic salt and/or coarse sea salt

▸ In a medium saucepan, bring salted water to a boil and add the edamame. Return to a boil, then lower heat to maintain a slow rolling boil for 5 minutes, until warmed through. Watch carefully so that the boiling water does not foam up and overflow.

▸ Drain the edamame in a colander, then sprinkle liberally with salt and/or garlic salt. Serve cold or at room temperature. Don't eat the pods.

GOBBLIN' FINGERS

Radishes make creepy-looking fingernails on these oddly orange fingers.

5 fingers make a fine serving	Easy Ranch Dip (page 106)
	Baby carrots
	Radishes

▸ Prepare the Easy Ranch Dip and refrigerate several hours or overnight.

▸ Wash the radishes and use a sharp paring knife to cut small oval slices from the sides. Use a small amount of dip to attach radish slices as "fingernails" onto the baby carrots. Serve the fingers by poking them, fingernails up, out of a container filled with a small layer of dip.

LITTLE VITAMIN B_{12}

Vegans, are you getting your B_{12}? Vitamin B_{12} is the only vitamin that is not reliably supplied by a plant-based diet and exposure to the sun. Because of this, vegetarians and vegans may have low stores of the vitamin.

The good news is that the crystalline form of B_{12} in vitamin supplements and cereals is actually more easily absorbed by our bodies than the B_{12} found in animal products. In fact, even some meat eaters have been found to be lacking in B_{12} and could benefit from supplementation. (Source: "Vegetarians, Older Folks Advised to Get Enough B_{12}," Amy Norton, Reuters Health, August 2005).

So stay healthy! Make sure Vitamin B_{12} is included in your diet. Many nondairy milks, cereals, and veggie meats are fortified with B_{12}, and B_{12} supplements are inexpensive and available at most health food and grocery stores. For more information I recommend the article "What Every Vegan Should Know about Vitamin B_{12}," by Jack Norris, RD, at veganhealth.org/articles/everyvegan.

GREG'S GRANOLA

Granola makes a fine crunchy snack at any time of day. Pack a small, sealed container of granola separately so it stays crunchy, then sprinkle it over soy yogurt and fresh fruit at lunchtime.

This is my husband's favorite granola; feel free to substitute your own favorite dried fruit or nuts.

Makes about
4 cups

3 cups old-fashioned rolled oats

$^1/_2$ cup chopped pecans

$^1/_2$ teaspoon nutmeg

$^3/_4$ teaspoon cinnamon

A pinch of salt

$^1/_4$ cup canola oil

$^1/_3$ cup maple syrup

$^1/_2$ cup diced dried apple

$^1/_2$ cup raisins

▸ Preheat the oven to 300°F.
▸ In a large mixing bowl, combine the oats, pecans, nutmeg, cinnamon, and salt. Stir with a large wooden spoon to combine.
▸ In a 2-cup liquid measuring cup or small bowl, whisk together the canola oil and maple syrup. Pour the liquid over the oat mixture, stirring well to coat the oats completely with the oil and syrup.
▸ Spread the mixture out evenly on a baking sheet and place in the oven. Bake until the granola is lightly toasted, about 30 minutes, stirring once halfway through. Remove from the oven and place the baking sheet on a wire rack to cool. Stir in the dried apple and raisins, then store in an airtight container.

LUNCH BOX FONDUE

My son loves this creamy, cheesy fondue. His favorite dippers are steamed brussels sprouts; he asks me for fondue every time he sees good-looking sprouts at the store. This recipe also makes a nice "cheese" sauce to pour over baked potatoes or steamed greens.

Makes about 2 cups

½ cup sliced baby carrots

1 (12-ounce) package soft or firm silken tofu

¼ cup nutritional yeast flakes

¼ teaspoon dry mustard

1 tablespoon mellow white miso

1 teaspoon freshly squeezed lemon juice

¾ teaspoon salt (or to taste)

A pinch of white pepper

A pinch of nutmeg

▸ Place the carrots in a small saucepan and cover with a scant ½ cup of water. Bring to boil and lower the heat to a simmer. Cook until the carrots are completely tender.

▸ Meanwhile, place all the rest of the ingredients in a blender. When the carrots are done add them and their cooking liquid and puree until completely smooth.

▸ Place the fondue back into the saucepan and heat on medium-low heat, stirring frequently, until piping hot.

▸ To serve immediately, pour the fondue into a small slow cooker or fondue pot and serve surrounded by vegetables and bread for dipping (our list of favorites follows).

▸ To pack fondue for a lunch, pour the hot fondue into a small insulated food jar that has been preheated with boiling water for 10 minutes.

Some favorite fondue dippers:

- cubes of crusty whole-grain bread
- boiled baby new potatoes
- lightly steamed baby carrots
- raw or lightly steamed cauliflower florets
- raw or lightly steamed broccoli florets
- steamed brussels sprouts
- blanched asparagus spears
- bell pepper strips
- apple chunks
- cherry tomatoes
- artichoke hearts
- raw button mushrooms
- raw zucchini slices
- blanched whole green beans
- pineapple chunks
- baby corn
- pickled jalapeños
- large, pitted olives
- celery sticks
- a spoon!

PICKY EATERS

My son HATES cooked leafy greens. Spinach, cabbage, kale, chard, collards, you name it—the sight of a stray bit of cooked leafy on his plate is enough to send him into hysterics. He also hates most dried fruit, winter squash, sweet potatoes, mushrooms, onions, hot cereal, cold cereal, plums, eggplant, bell peppers . . . could I ever go on! Sometimes he simply refuses to eat anything at all.

But is he a picky eater? I wouldn't say so. He loves broccoli, green beans, brussels sprouts, and cauliflower, and he's never met a lima bean he didn't like. He's also usually willing to try a new food at least once before making a face.

Aren't we all—kids and adults alike—picky eaters in our own way? I could create a list of likes and dislikes similar to the one above for my husband or myself. We each grew up with foods we loved and foods we couldn't stand. Some of our tastes changed as we grew; some stayed the same (my stepdad is still waiting for me to like green bell pepper so he can consider me officially grown up).

Our taste buds like what they like, regardless of what others would wish us to eat. Too much pressure on children to eat something they really don't like can backfire, leading to a stubborn, rebellious refusal to try anything new at all.

If your child has tried a food a few times and still doesn't like it, don't make her eat it. For example, although you will find onions are called for in some of my recipes, because James hates onions with such passion, I make all my recipes without onions when I make them for him. Feel free to leave onions or anything else your child will take exception to out of a recipe.

Mealtimes should be relaxed and enjoyable for everyone. If you fill your house with a wide variety of healthy choices, limit unhealthy foods, get regular checkups, and offer appropriate supplements (such as calcium-fortified beverages, iron-fortified cereal, and a chewable vegan multivitamin), everything should be okay. Here are a few more tips:

- Experiment, trying new foods together. My uncle used to take his young grandchildren to the grocery store each Saturday morning and would ask them to pick one new fruit or vegetable to try that day. Some they liked, some they didn't, but the point was to have fun. If you explore healthy foods with the same sense of adventure, you may be surprised at what your child enjoys.

- If a particular fruit or vegetable is turned down in one dish, try serving it another way—raw instead of cooked, or roasted instead of steamed. Try chopping or shredding it into tinier, kid-size bites (some kids are more bothered by the size of those big pieces of lettuce in the salad rather than their actual taste). Or try using a blender to puree it into velvety soups and smoothies.

- Don't give up too soon. Experts say children usually need to be presented with a new food several times before they will accept it. Try bringing back old rejects for another try later on. James abhorred cooked tomatoes until he turned seven. One day he smelled some Roasted Tomato Basil Soup (page 121) bubbling on the stove. "Do you think I'd like that?" he asked. I stifled my immediate response ("No, you don't like tomatoes") and said, "Maybe. It's very good soup." He ate three bowls for lunch! It taught me that a kid's tastes are his own, and there is always, always hope.

Except when it comes to me and green peppers, of course.

MINI WELLINGTONS

The day I discovered that Pepperidge Farm puff pastry sheets are vegan, there was much rejoicing and dancing in the store aisles. I've always been a sucker for anything *en croûte* (wrapped in pastry).

These are wonderful as is, but if you like mushrooms, check out the variation on page 78.

Makes 12 Mini Wellingtons

1 cup walnuts

1 cup cooked brown rice

1 cup canned chickpeas, rinsed and drained

1 cup oat bran

$\frac{1}{2}$ teaspoon sage

$\frac{1}{2}$ teaspoon marjoram

$\frac{1}{4}$ teaspoon thyme

$\frac{1}{4}$ teaspoon onion powder

2 tablespoons soy sauce

1 tablespoon Dijon mustard

1 tablespoon natural peanut butter

1 (1-pound) package frozen puff pastry, thawed at room temperature for about 30 minutes

Extra virgin olive oil, for brushing

▸ Line two baking sheets with parchment paper, spray with non-stick spray, and set aside. Have a small bowl of water and a clean, floured pastry board or flat surface ready.

▸ Using a food processor fitted with the S blade, process the walnuts into very small bits. Scrape the walnuts into a large mixing bowl and set aside.

▸ Add the brown rice and chickpeas to the bowl of the food processor and process until the mixture forms a coarse mash. Add this mash to the mixing bowl along with the oat bran, sage, marjoram, thyme, onion powder, soy sauce, mustard, and peanut butter. Using your hands, knead the mixture well until it is thoroughly mixed and holds its shape. Cool completely (if the filling is too warm it will melt the puff pastry and the pastry won't bake up puffy and crisp).

▸ Unfold the first sheet of puff pastry on a floured pastry board or flat surface (it should still be cold, but thawed enough to unfold without cracking). Using a rolling pin, roll the pastry out into a 12 x 12-inch square. Cut the sheet into six rectangles, each about 6 x 4 inches.

▸ Scoop up a handful of the nut loaf mixture and form it into a small rectangular loaf, about 3 x 1 x ¾ inches. Place the loaf in the center of a piece of puff pastry. Dip your fingers in the bowl of water and lightly wet the top of the loaf.

▸ Fold the short ends of the puff pastry up over the loaf, then fold the long edges up, using a bit of water on the edges of the pastry to help seal it shut. The loaf should be completely encased in puff pastry.

▸ Place the Mini Wellingtons, seam side down, on the prepared baking sheets. Repeat with the other sheet of puff pastry and the remaining bean and nut mixture. Lightly brush the pastries with olive oil.

▸ You may score the tops of the puff pastry with a decorative design using a very sharp knife or razor blade. Don't cut completely through the puff pastry.

▸ Cover the baking sheets completely with plastic wrap and refrigerate overnight or until ready to bake.

▸ When ready to bake, preheat the oven to 400°F (give the oven plenty of time to warm up to ensure a good puff pastry crust). Bake for 25 minutes, until the crust is puffed and golden and the inside is heated through.

VARIATION: We adults love this version with mushrooms: Sauté 2 cups minced button mushrooms, 1 minced garlic clove, and a pinch of salt in 2 teaspoons olive oil over medium-high heat until the moisture has evaporated and the mushrooms are soft, fragrant, and starting to brown, about 5 minutes. Stir the mushrooms into the nut loaf mixture and proceed with the recipe.

VARIATION: Stuffed Peppers: My lovely sister-in-law devised this healthy variation made without the puff pastry: "I made the nut and bean loaf, then added a ¼ cup of tomato sauce. I stuffed it into seven cleaned-out medium green bell peppers and baked them at 350°F for 30 minutes. They tasted great, travel nicely (I took one to work), and are very filling! While I was stuffing the peppers, I noticed that (for me) cutting a slit down one of the sides is helpful in stuffing the pepper, but you might be better at stuffing than I am." Thanks, Rachel!

MUSUBI

These rice balls were a favorite snack of my Japanese uncle, who loved to eat them with the traditional *umeboshi* filling. Umeboshi are tart, salty, pickled plums, and you may find them to be a bit of an acquired taste.

If pickled plum is too much of a stretch for your little luncher, Japanese schoolchildren have also started enjoying their musubi with a new filling: peanut butter!

Makes 6 musubi,
serves 3

----
2 cups uncooked Japanese sticky rice

Kosher or sea salt

Nori seaweed, cut into strips or squares

6 pitted umeboshi (or 6 teaspoons natural
    peanut butter)

▸ Cook the sticky rice according to package directions, or as follows: rinse and drain the rice, then place in a medium saucepan with 2½ cups water (1 part rice to 1¼ parts water). Bring to a boil and set the heat to low. Cover and cook on low for 25 minutes, until the water is absorbed and the rice is tender. Uncover and toss the rice with a rice paddle or wooden spoon, then allow to cool.

▸ Meanwhile, have a bowl of water, a salt shaker, nori strips, and your filling ingredients ready.

▸ When the rice is cool enough to handle, moisten your hands with water, then sprinkle some salt on your palms. Spoon up a large ball of rice, about the size of a racquet ball, and use your hands to press the rice into a ball or triangle.

▸ Push your thumb into the center of the rice, fill with one pitted umeboshi plum or a teaspoon of peanut butter, and cover the hole with rice. Set the musubi on a strip or square of nori. Use a bit of water on your fingertips to moisten the nori so it will stick, then wrap it around the musubi.

▶ Cover the rice balls with plastic wrap until lunchtime.

VARIATION: Last Easter we shaped our musubi into "eggs" and decorated them with colorful soy paper (*mamenori*) to make vegan Easter Eggs. Place the filling where the egg yolk would be!

NATIVE BLEND POPCORN BALLS

You might consider bringing this treat into the classroom to share. As the students munch away, you can share with them that popcorn, sunflowers, pumpkins, blueberries, and cranberries were used by the Native Americans and are all foods native to our continent (see page 57). They're darn tasty, too!

Makes 12 balls

$1/3$ cup roasted, unsalted pumpkin seeds
    (or buy them raw and toast your own,
    see below)
10 cups popped popcorn ($1/2$ cup unpopped
    kernels, popped in $1/8$ cup corn or
    canola oil)
$1/3$ cup roasted, unsalted sunflower seeds
$1/3$ cup dried blueberries
$1/3$ cup dried cranberries
$1/4$ cup brown rice syrup
1 cup packed light brown sugar
$1/2$ teaspoon salt
Margarine or oil for hands

- To toast raw pumpkin seeds, preheat the oven to 350°F. Place the pumpkin seeds on a baking sheet and toast, shaking the pan one or two times, for 10 minutes, until the seeds are slightly puffed. Set aside.

- Pop the popcorn and place it in a large mixing bowl with the sunflower seeds, pumpkin seeds, dried blueberries, and dried cranberries. Remove any unpopped kernels. Set aside.

- Place the brown rice syrup, brown sugar, salt, and ¼ cup water in a small saucepan over medium heat. Cook, stirring constantly, until the mixture boils over the entire surface. Stop stirring and adjust the heat if necessary to maintain this constant boil without boiling over.

- Okay, now you have a choice. If you want soft, somewhat gooey, chewy popcorn balls (my personal preference), boil for about 8 to 10 minutes (240°F on a candy thermometer, also known as soft-ball stage). If you want hard, less chewy popcorn balls that crackle when you crunch into them (my husband's preference), boil for up to 15 minutes (250°F on a candy thermometer, or hard-ball stage).

- Pour the sugar mixture evenly over the popcorn, stirring constantly until everything is completely coated, being sure to stir from the bottom of the bowl to catch all those little sunflower seeds that like to fall to the bottom. Put some margarine or oil on your hands to keep the mixture from sticking. Scoop up large handfuls and shape into balls, pressing firmly (if you are packing some inside a lunch box, make sure you make them small or flat enough so that they fit with the lid closed).

- Work quickly before the mixture has a chance to cool. If the mixture gets too firm to shape, place it in a warm (300°F) oven for 1 to 2 minutes to soften.

PERFECT PEPITAS

Pepitas (green pumpkin seeds) are available in bulk bins at most health foods stores and some grocery stores. They are an excellent source of protein, iron, and other minerals. These savory, smoky pumpkin seeds are reminiscent of bacon bits. Use them as a garnish on salads, soups, and greens, or eat them by the handful for a high-protein snack.

Makes 1 cup

---

1 cup raw, hulled pepitas

A large pinch (about $1/16$ teaspoon) cayenne

1 tablespoon Bragg Liquid Aminos
   (or soy sauce)

$1/2$ teaspoon liquid smoke flavoring

▸ Heat a large cast-iron skillet over medium heat. Place the pumpkin seeds in the skillet and stir constantly with a wooden spoon. Toast the seeds for about 8 to 10 minutes, until the seeds are puffed and making popping noises. Lower the heat as needed to avoid burning; some of the seeds should turn a golden brown.

▸ Remove from heat and sprinkle with the cayenne. Pour in the Liquid Aminos or soy sauce and the liquid smoke (the liquid should sizzle when it hits the pan—don't inhale that first puff of peppery smoke!). Return the skillet to the burner, stirring continually. Stir and scrape the bottom of the skillet until the seeds are dry, about 1 to 2 minutes.

▸ Pour the seeds out onto a large plate and spread them out to cool. Cool completely and store in an airtight jar at room temperature.

PLAY PRETZELS

Don't even think about making Play Pretzels without some little hands around to help you! Get creative and have fun!

Makes about 3 dozen pretzels, depending on the size you make them

½ cup warm water (110°F)

1 teaspoon sugar

1 scant tablespoon (1 package) active dry yeast

⅔ cup whole wheat flour

⅔ cup all-purpose flour

¾ teaspoon kosher salt

Coarse salt or Perfect Cinnamon-Sugar (page 215), optional

▸ Preheat the oven to 425°F. Line two baking sheets with parchment paper, spray with nonstick spray, and set aside.

▸ Pour the warm water into a mug or liquid measuring cup and stir in the sugar. Sprinkle the yeast into the water and stir well. Let the mixture sit until it's bubbly and dissolved, about 5 minutes.

▸ Meanwhile, in a medium mixing bowl, whisk together the whole wheat flour, all-purpose flour, and salt. Pour the yeast mixture into the flour, stirring until a dough forms.

▸ Turn the dough out onto a lightly floured surface and knead for about 2 minutes, until a smooth dough forms. Cover the dough with plastic wrap and set aside to rest for 10 minutes.

▸ Pinch or cut off bits of the dough and roll into long, thin snakes, about ¼ inch wide. Form the snakes into letters, numbers, squares, spirals, pretzels, hearts, or other fun shapes.

▸ Place the shapes on the prepared baking sheet. Brush the pretzels with water using a pastry brush. If you like, sprinkle them with some coarse salt or Perfect Cinnamon-Sugar. Bake for about 10 minutes, until lightly golden.

POLENTA FRIES

Polenta is a coarse grind of cornmeal similar to grits. It is usually yellow, but white polenta and grits also make great fries.

The polenta is prepared the night before and refrigerated. In the morning allow about 20 minutes to slice and broil the polenta wedges, turning them into perfect, crispy fries. Instead of cooking your own polenta, you can use a tube of precooked polenta from the store. Slice and broil it into fries using the instructions above.

Makes 2 to 3 servings

4 cups water, lightly salted

1 ½ cups polenta or grits

1 tablespoon extra virgin olive oil, plus more for pan

1 tablespoon nutritional yeast flakes

Salt (optional)

Barbecue sauce or ketchup, for serving

▸ Spray or brush one 8.5 x 3.5-inch loaf pan with olive oil. Cut a piece of parchment paper large enough to cover the bottom of the loaf pan with two edges folding up and over the sides of the pan (this will help you unmold the polenta). Spray or brush the parchment paper with olive oil. Set aside.

▸ In a medium saucepan, bring the salted water to a boil. Gradually add the polenta, whisking constantly. Return to a boil, lower the heat to the lowest setting, and cook, stirring constantly with a wooden spoon, until the mixture is thick, about 8 minutes. Add the olive oil and the nutritional yeast and stir well to combine.

▸ Pour the polenta mixture into the prepared loaf pan. Use a wooden spoon or spatula to smooth the top. Refrigerate several hours or overnight.

▸ In the morning, preheat the oven to broil with the oven rack set about 5 to 6 inches from the broiler. Line a baking sheet with parchment paper and brush the paper with olive oil.

▸ Remove the polenta from the loaf pan and set it on a cutting board. Slice the polenta width-wise into ½-inch slices, then cut the slices in half to make bite-size pieces. Arrange the slices on the baking sheet and brush them with olive oil.

▸ Broil for about 10 minutes, until the tops are crispy. Flip the slices over and broil for an additional 5 minutes, until crispy and beginning to brown. Sprinkle with nutritional yeast flakes and/or salt if desired. Serve the fries with barbecue sauce or ketchup for dipping.

RAW VEGGIE SHAPES

Some raw vegetables can be cut into fun shapes for snacking or dipping. Sweet, crunchy jicama is our favorite, but many different raw veggies work nicely. Use a mix of different vegetables for a variety of colors.

Makes 1 to several servings

Special equipment you will need:
Small, sharp cookie cutters (preferably metal)

One or more raw vegetables:
Jicama
Kohlrabi
Daikon radish
Large carrots
Sweet potato/yam
Golden beets

- Peel your veggies and slice them into thin circles (about ⅛ inch thick).
- Use small, sharp cookie cutters to cut out decorative shapes. Press down evenly and firmly. Save the scraps to chop up and add to salad later on.

VARIATION: Try using long strips taken from the sides of zucchini, cucumber, or tomatoes. Keep the skin on to help the veggies hold together.

SWEET POTATO OVEN FRIES

If you are used to eating sweet potatoes candied with brown sugar and cinnamon, you might be surprised to discover how good they can be with savory seasonings like olive oil, garlic, or onions. Roasting brings out their flavor and turns them into a great substitute for regular french fries.

Makes 2 servings

One large sweet potato or red garnet yam, peeled and cut into 2½ x ½ x ½-inch fries (about 3 cups)
1 teaspoon extra virgin olive oil
¼ teaspoon garlic salt
Salt (optional)

- Preheat the oven to 475°F. Line a baking sheet with parchment paper and set aside.
- In a medium bowl, toss together the sweet potatoes, olive oil, and garlic salt. Spread in a single layer on the baking sheet.
- Roast the fries for about 20 minutes, stirring two or three times during the roasting to ensure even cooking. Watch them carefully

toward the end of roasting so they don't burn; they should be cooked through and golden brown. Salt to taste and serve.

VARIATION: For a real grown-up treat, try topping these sweet potato fries with red onion slices browned in olive oil.

TOFU APPLE SPRING ROLLS

My husband tells me this recipe is worth the entire price of the book! Tofu is baked in a flavorful orange-ginger marinade, then paired with tart apple and sweet Napa cabbage and rolled in a rice paper wrapper. For younger kids, try leaving out the cabbage, cilantro, and scallion. Serve with Quick Peanut Sauce (page 108) for dipping.

Makes 9 rolls

----
1 pound firm tofu

4 tablespoons freshly squeezed orange juice

1 tablespoon mirin (sweet Japanese cooking wine)

1 tablespoon soy sauce

1 tablespoon canola oil

2 garlic cloves, minced

1 tablespoon minced fresh ginger

A pinch of cayenne

1 Granny Smith apple

9 (8-inch diameter) dried rice paper wrappers (see note on page 49)

18 fresh cilantro stems

1 cup finely shredded Napa cabbage

1 bunch scallions, sliced

9 large leaf or butterhead lettuce leaves, washed and patted dry
----

- Wrap the tofu in a kitchen towel and set it on a plate. Put another plate on top and weigh it down with something heavy. Press the tofu for 30 minutes.
- Make a marinade by whisking together 3 tablespoons of the orange juice, the mirin, soy sauce, and canola oil. Stir in the garlic, ginger, and cayenne.
- Cut the tofu into three slices lengthwise, then turn the tofu block on its side and cut into thirds again, making nine equal slices. Place the slices in an 8 x 8-inch baking dish and pour the marinade over the top. Let the tofu sit for 30 minutes, then turn the slices over and let sit for another 30 minutes.
- Preheat the oven to 375°F. Bake the tofu and marinade for 40 minutes, until it is golden brown and the marinade is absorbed. Set aside to cool.
- Peel, core, and thinly slice the Granny Smith apple. Toss the apple slices with the remaining tablespoon of orange juice to keep them from browning.
- Dip one of the wrappers in a wide bowl filled with warm water for 15 seconds, or until softened. Transfer to a dry work surface and pat dry. Arrange a slice of tofu along with some apple slices, 2 sprigs of cilantro, some Napa cabbage, and scallions in a mound just below the center of the wrapper. Roll up the rice paper to form a tight bundle, folding in the sides along the way.
- Serve or pack each roll wrapped in a lettuce leaf (this will keep the spring roll from sticking to the plate). If packing for later, cover the rolls with a damp paper towel and some plastic wrap to keep them from drying out.

TOFU LETTUCE CUPS WITH MANGO CHUTNEY

The mix of lively flavors sings in the mouth with every bite of these easy-to-make lettuce cups!

In this recipe the tofu is steam-fried, which infuses it with the fresh ginger and soy sauce without using any oil. Cook the tofu well ahead of time and refrigerate before assembling the lettuce cups.

Makes 18 lettuce cups

1 tablespoon minced fresh ginger

1 tablespoon soy sauce

2 tablespoons water, plus more as needed

1 pound firm tofu, drained and cut into 18 cubes

1 large head butterhead lettuce, leaves separated, washed, and patted dry

Approximately ½ cup roasted peanuts, coarsely chopped

Approximately 1 tablespoon toasted coconut

1 lime

1 jar mango chutney

▶ Heat a nonstick or cast-iron skillet over medium-high heat. Stir together the minced ginger, soy sauce, and water. Pour the mixture into the hot pan; the liquid should sizzle and begin to bubble. Add the tofu cubes in a single layer and cook, turning frequently, until the tofu is touched with brown and warmed through and all the liquid has been cooked off (turn down the heat and add a bit more water if the liquid is boiling off too fast).

▶ Remove the tofu cubes from the pan and place on a platter in the refrigerator to chill for several hours.

- To assemble the lettuce cups, lay out the lettuce leaves so that they curl upward. Sprinkle each leaf with a generous teaspoon of chopped peanuts and about $\frac{1}{4}$ teaspoon coconut (use more or less as desired). Top each leaf with a tofu cube and sprinkle with a generous squeeze of fresh lime juice.
- Top each tofu cube with a dollop of mango chutney, or serve chutney on the side.
- To eat, pick up a lettuce cup with your fingers and fold the lettuce around the filling slightly like a taco shell. Try to get a bit of tofu, chutney, peanuts, and coconut in every bite.

SALADS AND DRESSINGS

"AND THEN, A MIRACLE OCCURRED. . . "

Thursday, Nov. 3, 2005: *Tonight my son* ATE A SALAD! *I saw it happen! I can't believe it—the same kid who objected to even a wayward bit of ice-berg lettuce on a bite of burrito suddenly ate his greens!*

James had wandered into the kitchen and was watching me chop lettuce and spinach. He picked up a baby spinach leaf, examined it, and handed it to me. "I think I could eat that if it had a yummy dress-ing on it," he told me, "and if it had things I like in it, like carrots."

WHAT?!? Okay, I thought, I must show no emotion, lest I spook the strange creature and cause it to flee. "Sure, I think we can do that," I calmly replied. I put him to work spinning the lettuce and chopping chunks of carrot and apple while I tried to come up with a "yummy dressing."

I had to think fast. Suddenly, I remembered a recent podcast on salad dressing by vegan cookbook author Dreena Burton. I hastily pulled out my notes. She suggested adding a sweetener, like maple

continues

syrup, to cut acidity. Starting with her example, I put together a dressing I am now calling Asian Miracle Dressing.

Together we brought the salad of greens, carrots, apple, walnuts, and dressing to the table, and I served my son up a bowlful.

"Mmm, this dressing is my number one dressing!" he said as he started in.

"So many flavors!" he said a few bites later.

He ate two bowlfuls.

I tried not to gape. The immutable law of Green Leafy Hatred had suddenly and inexplicably reversed itself!

ASIAN MIRACLE DRESSING

(Results atypical; individual results may vary; please try this at home.)

Makes approximately ½ cup

2 tablespoons balsamic vinegar

¼ teaspoon Dijon mustard

1 ½ tablespoons maple syrup

A pinch of salt

A grind of pepper

½ teaspoon soy sauce

1 teaspoon toasted sesame oil

1 ½ tablespoons extra virgin olive oil

▸ Combine all ingredients and whisk with a fork until well blended.

ASIAN SALAD WITH ORANGE SESAME DRESSING

This recipe is designed to create two individually arranged salads. If it's easier for you, toss all the salad ingredients together in a single bowl and serve with dressing on the side, or arrange them into several smaller salads.

Makes 2 large salads

Dressing:
¼ cup freshly squeezed orange juice
    (the juice of one orange)
¼ cup brown rice vinegar
1 teaspoon toasted sesame oil
Salt
Shichimi togarashi (Japanese seven-spice
    blend) if you have it, or cayenne.

▸ Combine orange juice, brown rice vinegar, and toasted sesame oil. Season to taste with salt and shichimi togarashi and set aside.

Salad:
1 (5-ounce) bag of spring mix or baby
    lettuce salad greens
¾ cup carrot, peeled and grated,
    loosely packed
¾ cup daikon radish, peeled and grated,
    loosely packed
1 cup cucumber, peeled and diced
1 cup shelled edamame, thawed if frozen
Toasted sesame seeds

▸ Arrange the salad greens in a small mound on each of two salad plates. Mix together the grated carrot and daikon radish and arrange around the edges of each bed of lettuce, forming a wreath. Mix together the cucumber and edamame and place half in the center of each lettuce bed. Sprinkle the cucumber mixture with toasted sesame seeds. Add the dressing just before serving.

CHICKPEA SALAD

This luscious salad makes a great sandwich filling tucked into a whole wheat pita with lettuce and spinach, or it can be enjoyed on its own as a side dish or on top a bed of mixed greens.

Use roasted chickpeas for a chewier texture (roast them the night before to save time in the morning) or use them straight from the can if you're in a hurry.

Makes 2 servings

1 recipe Cheesy Roasted Chickpeas
(page 194), cooled, or Fast Cheesy
Chickpeas (page 194)
2 tablespoons Vegenaise
1 teaspoon toasted sesame oil
1 tablespoon minced fresh cilantro
2 tablespoons chopped pecans
1 celery stalk, minced
One scallion, white and part of the green,
minced (optional)

▸ Combine the chickpeas, Vegenaise, toasted sesame oil, cilantro, pecans, celery, and scallion in a medium bowl and mix gently with a spatula.

CUCUMBER RAITA

A *raita* is a cooling yogurt salad made with cucumber, tomato, onion, or grated carrot. According to Julie Sahni, author of *Classic Indian Cooking*, "an Indian meal, especially a vegetarian meal, is never considered complete without a dish containing yogurt."

Unfortunately, plain soy yogurt is not available in most areas, and even when it is, it can contain large amounts of sweetener, making it ill suited to a dish like raita. Here, I have substituted silken tofu. If you do have access to unsweetened plain soy yogurt—or better yet, if you make your own—use it in place of the silken tofu and lemon juice.

Makes 4 servings

1 medium-size cucumber

3/4 cup soft silken tofu

2 teaspoons freshly squeezed lemon juice
   (or more, to taste)

1/4 cup vegan sour cream (or more silken tofu)

A pinch of sugar

1/2 teaspoon kosher salt (or to taste)

1/2 teaspoon canola oil

1/4 teaspoon black mustard seeds

A pinch of asafoetida powder (optional)

▸ Peel the cucumber, trim off the ends, and cut in half lengthwise. Use a melon baller or teaspoon to scoop out the seeds. Grate the cucumber into a small bowl, using the large holes of a hand grater, and set aside.

▸ In a blender, combine the silken tofu, lemon juice, vegan sour cream, sugar, and salt. Puree until smooth. Pour over the cucumber and stir to combine.

▸ In a small, heavy skillet, heat the oil over medium-high heat. When the oil is hot, add the black mustard seeds and asafoetida powder, if desired. Cover the skillet with a lid and listen for the seeds to start popping. When they have begun to pop, scrape the oil and spices into the cucumber raita and stir well. Chill for an hour or so before serving. Taste for seasoning and add more lemon juice as needed to brighten the flavors.

EASY POTATO SALAD

Finally! It's the potato salad I longed for as a child—all the delicious potatoes and creamy dressing without the dreaded bits of raw onion and bell pepper. My son hates onions the same I way I used to (how soon we forget the picky palates of our youth!), so he's very happy to get this onion-free dish in his lunch box.

This salad is especially easy to throw together if you have leftover cooked potatoes in the fridge, but freshly cooked potatoes will absorb more of the flavor.

Makes 2 servings

2 medium-size new potatoes, boiled until
   tender but still holding their shape
$\frac{1}{2}$ teaspoon white vinegar
$\frac{1}{8}$ cup Vegenaise
$\frac{1}{4}$ teaspoon Dijon mustard
$\frac{1}{8}$ teaspoon garlic salt
1 tablespoon capers, rinsed and drained
   (optional)
1 tablespoon diced celery (optional)
Salt and pepper

▸ When the potatoes are cool enough to handle, peel the skin off with the back of a knife. Dice the potatoes and place them in a small mixing bowl.

▸ Add the white vinegar, Vegenaise, Dijon mustard, and garlic salt and stir gently with a spatula until well combined. Add the capers and/or celery, if using, and season to taste with salt and pepper.

FENNEL CUCUMBER SALAD

Fennel bulbs are licorice-flavored vegetables that are at their prime during the fall and winter months. Fennel bulbs can be roasted, grilled, sautéed, or eaten raw. Here, they are shaved paper-thin using a mandoline (an adjustable-blade slicer used to cut fruits and vegetables), then tossed with cucumber, capers, lemon, and olive oil.

Makes 4 servings

1 large fennel bulb, rinsed

$1/2$ medium-size cucumber

4 tablespoons capers, drained

$1/2$ teaspoon fresh lemon zest

1 tablespoon freshly squeezed lemon juice

$1/2$ teaspoon kosher salt (or to taste)

1 tablespoon extra virgin olive oil

Pitted Kalamata or black olives (optional)

▸ Cut the stalks off the fennel bulb, cutting close to the bulb. Remove any bruised or tough outer layers. Cut away the bottom of the bulb, then cut the bulb in half lengthwise and remove the hard inner core. Slice the fennel into paper-thin strips using a mandoline or vegetable slicer. If you don't have a mandoline, slice the fennel as thinly as possible with a large chef's knife.

▸ Peel the cucumber and rinse. Cut the cucumber into 2-inch pieces. If using a mandoline, adjust the blade to make matchsticks and cut the cucumber, rotating it to cut all around the outside, discarding the inner core of seeds. If slicing the cucumber by hand, cut the cucumber in half and scoop out the seeds, then cut into 2-inch-long matchsticks.

▸ Toss the fennel and cucumber together with the capers and lemon zest. In a small bowl, mix together the lemon juice, salt, and olive oil. Pour over the salad and toss well. Garnish each serving with one or two pitted olives.

GREEN BEANS AND CARROTS IN A TARRAGON VINAIGRETTE

The flavors of lemon and tarragon nicely complement the green beans and carrots in this simple salad. Double or triple the recipe to suit your needs. This vinaigrette also tastes lovely on boiled new potatoes or cooked beets.

Makes 1 serving

3 baby carrots, cut into matchsticks

1 handful fresh French green beans, trimmed (about 3 ounces)

1/2 teaspoon Dijon mustard

1/4 teaspoon salt (or to taste)

1 tablespoon freshly squeezed lemon juice

2 tablespoons extra virgin olive oil

1/2 teaspoon dried tarragon or 1 teaspoon fresh, minced

Freshly ground black pepper

▸ Bring a small saucepan of lightly salted water to a boil. Fill a mixing bowl with ice water set aside in the sink.

▸ When the water boils, add the carrot matchsticks and green beans. Boil until they are just tender and the beans are still bright green, about 4 minutes. Immediately drain off the boiling water and place the vegetables in the ice water bath (this stops the cooking and retains the bright color). Drain again and set aside.

▶ Meanwhile, make the vinaigrette: in a small measuring cup, whisk together the Dijon mustard, salt, and lemon juice with a fork. Slowly add the olive oil, whisking constantly. Add the tarragon and whisk to blend. Season to taste with black pepper.

▶ Drizzle the vegetables with a small amount of vinaigrette and toss gently.

HEART BEET SALAD

This has been a favorite Valentine's Day meal for my sweetie and me for several years now. The sweet flavor of the roasted beets marries beautifully with the flavors of orange and apple. Use blood oranges if you can find them.

Makes 4 servings

Special equipment you will need:
A small, heart-shaped cookie cutter

3 large beets, scrubbed but not peeled
1 tablespoon balsamic vinegar
3 tablespoons extra virgin olive oil
3 or 4 fresh basil leaves, cut into thin ribbons
Salt and pepper
1 head of butterhead lettuce or heart of romaine, washed and dried
1 large handful baby spinach leaves, washed and dried
1 celery stalk, chopped
1 tart apple, peeled, cored, and chopped
2 oranges (preferably blood oranges)
$1/4$ cup raw or toasted walnuts, chopped

- Preheat the oven to 450°F. Wrap the beets in foil or parchment paper and place on the oven rack. Roast the beets until they're tender when pierced with a sharp knife through their thickest part, about 60 to 75 minutes. Set aside to cool completely.
- Meanwhile, prepare the dressing: whisk together the balsamic vinegar, olive oil, and basil leaves. Season to taste with salt and pepper. Set aside.
- When the beets have cooled, use the back of a paring knife to peel off the outer skins. Lay each beet on its side and cut it into ¼-inch slices. Use the cookie cutter to make heart-shaped cutouts (save the scraps to snack on or use in another dish).
- Cut or tear the lettuce into bite-size pieces, then place the lettuce, baby spinach, celery, and apple into a large salad bowl. Cut the orange in half and score as you would a grapefruit, then spoon out the orange segments into the bowl. Squeeze the remaining orange juice into the dressing and whisk to combine.
- To serve immediately, toss the salad with the dressing, then arrange on plates topped with the heart beets and walnuts. If packing for a lunch, arrange the beets and walnuts on top of the salad in a lunch container, with a smaller container of dressing on the side.

NITER KEBBEH (SPICE-INFUSED OIL)

Niter Kebbeh is the foundation flavor for Ethiopian stews; it is traditionally made with clarified butter, but mild canola oil works nicely. In addition to using it in Ethiopian recipes, you can also add a drizzle of this oil to soups, stews, cooked beans, or steamed mixed vegetables for a dash of exotic aroma and flavor.

Makes about
½ cup

½ cup canola oil

¼ onion, chopped into large pieces

2 garlic cloves, peeled and crushed

2 slices (¼-inch) fresh ginger

¼ teaspoon turmeric

2 cardamom pods, crushed

1 clove

1 (2-inch) cinnamon stick

A pinch of nutmeg

▸ Combine all the ingredients in a small saucepan. Bring to a simmer; reduce the heat to very low and simmer for 10 minutes, stirring occasionally. Let the oil sit for another 20 minutes to allow the flavors to develop. Strain the oil through a fine mesh sieve and store in the refrigerator.

PETITE PASTA SALAD

This is a fun and easy way to showcase the small star or alphabet pasta shapes commonly used in vegetable soup.

James usually doesn't like pasta salad; he says it is "too sour." I think the amount of vinegar in most commercial dressings is too strong for his taste. So I took it easy here and added just a touch of white vinegar mixed with white balsamic vinegar, which is mellower and sweeter than plain balsamic vinegar. Adjust the seasonings and vegetables according to your taste.

Makes 4 to 6 servings

1 (7-ounce) package tiny star or alphabet pasta
1 cup frozen corn
8 ounces sugar snap or snow peas, cut into bite-size pieces
1 cucumber (peeled or not, as desired), cut into bite-size pieces
1 tomato, seeded and diced
1/2 a red or orange bell pepper, diced
1 (2.25-ounce) can sliced black olives, rinsed and drained
1/2 cup chopped fresh cilantro
1 tablespoon chopped fresh basil
2 tablespoons extra virgin olive oil
1 to 2 tablespoons white wine vinegar (or to taste)
1 teaspoon white balsamic vinegar
Salt and white pepper

▶ Bring a medium-size saucepan of water to a boil. Add the pasta and cook until just barely tender, about 2 to 3 minutes. During the last minute, add the frozen corn and chopped sugar snap or snow peas.

▸ Drain the pasta, corn, and peas and rinse well with cold running water. Drain.

▸ In a large mixing bowl, toss the pasta, corn, and peas with the rest of the vegetables and fresh herbs.

▸ In a small bowl whisk together the olive oil and vinegars and season to taste with salt and white pepper. Pour over the pasta salad and toss together until well combined. Taste and adjust seasonings as needed.

SPROUT SALAD WITH MANDARIN ORANGE DRESSING

Making your own sprouts for this salad is a great way to teach children about the life cycle of plants. Sprouting is a perfect activity for the early springtime, when the seeds that have been asleep in the soil all winter long are getting ready to burst forth with new life.

Makes 4 servings

1 can (11 ounces) mandarin orange segments

1 teaspoon maple syrup

1/8 cup white wine vinegar

1/2 teaspoon kosher salt (or to taste)

A pinch of freshly ground black pepper
  (or to taste)

A pinch of cayenne (or to taste)

1/8 cup canola oil

4 cups Homemade Sprouts (see page 197)

2 large carrots, peeled and grated

Butterhead lettuce

A small handful toasted, unsalted
  sunflower seeds

- Drain the canned mandarin orange segments, reserving ⅛ cup of the mandarin juice for the dressing. Set aside the orange segments to top the salad.
- To make the dressing, in a liquid measuring cup whisk together the mandarin orange juice, maple syrup, white wine vinegar, salt, pepper, and cayenne. Slowly whisk in the canola oil. Set aside.
- In a large salad bowl, combine the sprouts and grated carrot.
- To serve, line a plate or lunch box container with a lettuce leaf. Place a mound of the sprout mixture on the lettuce leaf, then top with mandarin orange segments and a sprinkle of sunflower seeds. Drizzle with the mandarin orange dressing just before serving.

DIPS, SAUCES, AND SPREADS

EASY HUMMUS

This is a simple, bare-bones recipe for hummus, without any of the green flecks of parsley or bits of raw garlic that sometimes turn children off.

Feel free to experiment with different types of beans or additional flavorings, like mellow white miso, fresh herbs, nutritional yeast, or ground nuts.

Makes about
2 cups

1 (15-ounce) can chickpeas, drained,
　　liquid reserved
1 tablespoon tahini (sesame paste)
2 tablespoons freshly squeezed lemon juice
1/4 teaspoon ground cumin
1/4 teaspoon paprika
1/2 teaspoon kosher salt (or to taste)
1 tablespoon extra virgin olive oil (optional)

- Combine all the ingredients and process in a food processor fitted with the S blade until completely smooth, stopping to scrape down the sides once or twice during processing.
- If your food processor has difficulty processing the beans or the mixture seems too dry, add a bit of the liquid from the can of beans, just enough to get the mixture going.
- Serve on bread or in pita for sandwiches or as a dip for baked pita chips, crackers, and veggies.

EASY RANCH DIP

This makes a fabulous dip for veggies, crackers, or baked potato crisps. Of course, you can always replace regular sour cream with vegan sour cream and use a ranch dressing mix (check the label—some contain dairy). We prefer this recipe using beans and soy "buttermilk" to replace the sour cream; it's delicious, lower in fat, and appeals to those of us who wish to avoid processed foods.

Makes about
2 cups

1/2 cup plain, unsweetened soymilk

1 tablespoon freshly squeezed lemon juice

1 (15-ounce) can white beans,
    rinsed and drained

1 teaspoon dried dill weed

1 teaspoon dried parsley

1/4 teaspoon dried tarragon

1/4 teaspoon onion powder

1/4 teaspoon garlic powder

A pinch of cayenne

1/2 teaspoon salt (or to taste)

Freshly ground black or white pepper

- Combine the soymilk and lemon juice and set aside for 2 minutes (the mixture will curdle). Add the soy "buttermilk" to the beans in a blender and blend on high until completely smooth, about 2 minutes or more, scraping down the sides of the blender as needed.
- Spoon the mixture into a bowl and stir in the rest of the ingredients, seasoning with pepper to taste. Cover and chill for several hours in the refrigerator before serving.

LAYERED BEAN DIP

Finally, a way to pack avocado in the lunch box so it won't turn brown! Enclosing the avocado in layers of bean dip keeps air out and prevents browning from oxidation.

Makes 2 servings

1 cup Refried Black Beans
    (page 203, or use canned refried beans)
½ cup salsa
1 ripe avocado
Freshly squeezed lemon or lime juice
Sea salt
Vegan sour cream (optional)
Black olives, pitted and sliced

- In a small bowl, mix the refried beans and salsa together.
- In another small bowl, scoop out the ripe avocado and mash with a fork. Add a squeeze of lemon or lime juice and sea salt to taste.
- Use a small spatula to spread a layer of the bean mixture at the bottom of your lunch container, then spread a layer of avocado mixture over the beans. Cover the avocado with another layer of beans (make sure the avocado is completely covered to avoid

discoloration). Top the beans with a layer of vegan sour cream, if desired, and decorate the top with olive slices.

▸ Serve with tortilla chips and veggies on the side for dipping.

VARIATION: Get creative and add more layers to your dip: shredded vegan cheese, chopped lettuce and/or tomato, or sliced green onions.

QUICK PEANUT SAUCE

A very simple and kid-friendly dipping sauce. Great with spring rolls or veggies, Quick Peanut Sauce is also lovely over cooked noodles.

Makes about
1 cup

½ cup natural peanut butter

1 teaspoon toasted sesame oil

2 tablespoons soy sauce

2 teaspoons golden brown sugar

1 tablespoon brown rice vinegar

1 clove garlic, finely minced

Tabasco pepper sauce

Salt

▸ In a small bowl, mix all ingredients together, seasoning with Tabasco and salt to taste. Slowly add ¼ to ½ cup of warm water or more to achieve desired consistency.

SNEAKY MOMMA'S TOMATO SAUCE

I finally found the way to get my family to eat kale—they have to be unaware that they are eating it! In this flavorful tomato sauce, the kale is not even noticeable. I like this sauce in its unblended state, with nice chunks of tomato and kale and carrot. But blend it smooth if you want to keep your secret safe.

Makes about 4 cups

1 tablespoon extra virgin olive oil

1/2 cup chopped onion

1/2 cup chopped red bell pepper (optional)

2 garlic cloves, minced

2 (28-ounce) cans whole peeled tomatoes, drained

1 (6-ounce) can tomato paste

1 cup shredded basil leaves

2 cups shredded kale leaves

1 large carrot, grated

2 tablespoons minced fresh parsley

1 teaspoon dried oregano

1/2 teaspoon dried thyme

A pinch of dried red pepper flakes

1/2 teaspoon sugar

1/2 teaspoon freshly ground black pepper

3/4 teaspoon salt (or to taste)

▶ Heat the olive oil in a wide saucepan over medium heat. Sauté the onion (and red bell pepper, if using) until soft, about 5 minutes. Add the garlic and sauté, stirring constantly, for 1 more minute.

▶ Add the tomatoes, tomato paste, basil, kale, carrot, parsley, oregano, thyme, and red pepper flakes. Break the whole tomatoes apart with the back of a wooden spoon and stir until everything is well blended. When the mixture begins to bubble, lower the heat and cook on low, stirring occasionally, for about one hour.

▸ Let cool slightly, then transfer the tomato sauce to a blender, working in batches if necessary. Blend until completely smooth, then transfer to a clean saucepan and stir over low heat until warm. Add the sugar, pepper, and salt.

▸ This tomato sauce also freezes well.

TOMATO ROSES ON A BED OF CANNELLINI BEAN PUREE

Finally, something worthwhile to do with those flavorless winter grocery store tomatoes! Their tight, unappetizing skin can be shaped into beautiful "roses" and nestled on top of a "long stem" of parsley as a cute, romantic garnish. The savory cannellini bean puree is made with rosemary-infused olive oil and garlic and served with crisp whole-grain crackers or pita chips.

Makes 4 servings

1 (15-ounce) can cannellini beans, rinsed and drained

1 1/2 teaspoons extra virgin olive oil

1 (4-inch) sprig of fresh rosemary

1 garlic clove, minced

1 tablespoon white wine vinegar

1/4 teaspoon salt (or to taste)

A pinch of white pepper (or to taste)

1 or 2 large, firm tomatoes

Italian parsley

▸ Rinse and drain the cannellini beans, then place them in the bowl of a food processor fitted with the S blade. Set aside.

▶ Heat the olive oil in a small skillet set over medium heat. When hot, add the rosemary sprig and cook, turning occasionally, until the rosemary is dark and limp and the oil is very aromatic, about 2 minutes. Remove the rosemary from the oil and discard. Add the garlic and cook, stirring constantly, until the garlic is soft, about 1 minute. Scrape the oil and garlic into the food processor and add the white wine vinegar, salt, and pepper. Process until completely smooth, stopping to scrape down the sides of the bowl as needed.

▶ To make the rose garnish, bring a small saucepan of water to a boil. Have a small bowl of ice water ready. Submerge the tomato in the boiling water for 30 seconds, then immediately plunge the tomato into cold water to stop the cooking. Dry off the tomato, then use a sharp paring knife to cut off two long, thin strips of tomato skin. Wrap the strips into tight spirals to form the roses.

▶ To serve, spoon the bean puree into a serving dish and use a spatula to smooth the top. Lay a large sprig of Italian parsley on the surface and nestle the tomato roses gently on top of the beans, surrounded by parsley leaves. Serve with crackers or pita crisps for dipping.

SOUPS AND STEWS

BROCCOLI FENNEL SOUP

This recipe uses the feathery fronds on the top of the fennel bulb. Save the bulb itself to use in the Roasted Vegetable Broth on page 123.

Makes 4 to 6
servings

----

1 large leek, trimmed and rinsed well

1 garlic clove, minced

1 teaspoon ground fennel seeds

1 tablespoon extra virgin olive oil

6 cups Roasted Vegetable Broth (page 123)
    or water

1/4 cup plus 1 tablespoon uncooked white rice

1 large head broccoli, cut into large florets
    (4–5 cups)

The feathery fronds from one fennel bulb,
    finely minced

1 teaspoon salt (or to taste)

Freshly ground black pepper (optional)

- Chop the leek into ½-inch pieces, using the white and lighter green part only, discarding the dark green top.
- In a large saucepan over medium heat, sauté the leek, garlic, and fennel seeds in the olive oil until soft, about 3 to 4 minutes. Add the stock or water and uncooked rice, bring to a boil, and simmer for 10 minutes. Add the broccoli and fennel fronds and simmer until the broccoli is completely tender, about 15 minutes.
- Working in batches if necessary, puree the soup in a blender until smooth. Pour the soup into a clean saucepan and add the salt. Add some freshly ground black pepper if desired. Serve immediately or pack into a preheated insulated food jar for lunch.

CREAMY CAULIFLOWER SOUP

This warm, golden cauliflower soup gets just a hint of cheesiness from nutritional yeast. The soup is filled with potatoes, carrots, and cauliflower—a great way to eat your vegetables!

Makes 6 cups

1 tablespoon extra virgin olive oil

½ a small onion, diced

1 large garlic clove, minced

1 ½ cups potato, peeled and chopped

1 cup peeled and diced carrots

1 small head cauliflower, cut into small florets
(about 6 cups)

1 ¼ teaspoons salt

¼ teaspoon white pepper (or more to taste)

1 tablespoon nutritional yeast flakes

- Heat the olive oil in a large saucepan over medium-high heat. Add the onion and sauté, stirring frequently, until the onion is soft and translucent, about 5 minutes. Add the garlic and cook, stirring, for another minute. Add the potatoes, carrots, and 4 cups of water. Bring to a boil and lower the heat. Simmer, covered, until the potatoes and carrots are completely tender (the potatoes should be falling-apart tender so the blended soup does not become gluey).

▸ Place the cauliflower florets in a steamer basket and steam until tender, about 10 minutes. Measure out 2 cups of the steamed cauliflower florets and set aside. Add the rest of the cauliflower to the potato mixture.

▸ Remove from heat and transfer the soup to a blender, in batches if necessary, and puree until smooth. Pour soup into a clean saucepan and return to the stove on medium-low heat. Add the cauliflower florets, salt, white pepper, and nutritional yeast flakes. Cook, stirring, until warmed through. Taste for salt and adjust as needed. Serve as is or sprinkle with Perfect Pepitas (page 82).

BEHOLD THE BLENDER

A good blender is one kitchen tool I consider absolutely essential. You'll need a good, high-quality blender for many of the recipes here, and quite frankly I would have a hard time being a parent without one.

Blending soups and sauces to a smooth consistency is a good way to make them more palatable to picky children. My son hates chunky sauces, or soups with several vegetables mixed together; he can't stop analyzing and fretting about what each little bit is. Blending leads to "out of sight, out of mind." I can tell him that an entire bunch of kale is in Sneaky Momma's Tomato Sauce (page 109), or that Sneaky Momma's Black Bean Soup (page 124) is filled with zucchini, bell pepper, and onions. As long he can't see them, he's okay with that.

I highly recommend you invest in the best blender you can possibly afford, and keep it out on the kitchen counter to blend kid-friendly smoothies and soups in a flash. Personally, I have used a Vita-Mix blender every day for over five years without ever having to replace a single part. Vita-Mix blenders are even strong enough to grind whole grains into fresh flour—*vroom!*

GOLDEN CHESTNUT SOUP

The first time we ever tried roasting chestnuts, my husband and I bought some on a whim at the grocery store ("Hey, look—chestnuts! Just like in that song!") We spread them out on a baking sheet and put them in the oven. Unfortunately, we didn't know you must cut a slit in the shell of the chestnut to release steam. In a few minutes, chestnuts were going off like fireworks, ricocheting inside the oven with deep, muffled booms. What a mess that was!

We learned our lesson that day, but we never gave up on chestnuts. They are delicious roasted and eaten plain as a snack, or pureed into a rich, golden soup.

Makes 4 servings

1 pound fresh chestnuts

4 large garlic cloves, unpeeled

1 tablespoon extra virgin olive oil

1 onion, chopped

1 carrot, diced

1 celery stalk, diced

4 sprigs fresh thyme

2 bay leaves

$^3/_4$ teaspoon salt (or to taste)

$^1/_8$ teaspoon nutmeg

$^1/_8$ teaspoon white pepper

▶ Preheat the oven to 475°F. Cut an "x" in the shell of each chestnut with a sharp paring knife. Arrange the chestnuts on a baking sheet with the unpeeled garlic cloves. Roast for 20 minutes, until the outer shell has pulled slightly away from the chestnut and the shell and inner skin peel away easily.

▶ Remove the outer shell and inner skin of each chestnut and place them in a bowl. Work quickly while the chestnuts are still hot (hold them with a kitchen towel if they are too hot to touch). Squeeze the roasted garlic out of the garlic cloves and add it to the bowl with the chestnuts. Set aside.

▸ In a medium saucepan, heat the olive oil over medium-high heat. Add the onion, carrot, celery, thyme, and bay leaves. Sauté, stirring often, until the onion is translucent, about 5 minutes. Add the chestnuts and garlic and 4 cups of water. Bring to a boil, lower the heat and simmer, covered, until the carrots are tender, about 10 minutes.

▸ Remove from heat. Remove the thyme sprigs and bay leaves and let the soup cool slightly. Transfer the soup to a blender, in batches if necessary, and puree until the soup is completely smooth. Pour the soup into a clean saucepan and add the salt, nutmeg, and white pepper. Warm over medium-low heat, stirring. Thin with water or broth as desired. Taste for salt and serve.

MASSUR DAL AND CARROT SOUP

In India, *dal* (split, hulled legumes or pulses) is a staple in the daily diet. A large portion of the population in India is vegetarian, and dal is an important and satisfying source of protein. In this dish, red lentils, known in India as massur dal, are cooked with carrots and pureed into a creamy, earthy soup.

Red lentils are lentils that have been hulled; do not substitute regular green or brown lentils.

Makes 6 servings

1 tablespoon canola oil
½ cup chopped onion
1 garlic clove, minced
½ teaspoon turmeric
1 teaspoon ground cumin

1 teaspoon ground coriander

1/8 teaspoon cayenne (or to taste), optional

1 cup uncooked red lentils, rinsed thoroughly
and drained

2 cups peeled and diced carrots

1 teaspoon sea salt

1 cup light coconut milk

1 tablespoon freshly squeezed lemon
or lime juice

▸ Heat the canola oil in a large saucepan over medium-high heat. Add the onion and sauté, stirring frequently, until the onion softens and just begins to brown, about 5 minutes. Add the garlic, turmeric, cumin, coriander, and cayenne (if using) and cook, stirring constantly, for another minute. Add the red lentils, carrots, and 4 cups water. Turn the heat to high, bring to a boil, then lower the heat and simmer, covered, until the carrots are completely tender and the lentils are dissolving, about 30 minutes. Allow the soup to cool slightly.

▸ Working in batches if necessary, pour the soup into a blender and blend until completely smooth. Transfer the pureed soup to a clean saucepan and return to the stove over low heat. Add the salt and coconut milk.

▸ Simmer for another 10 minutes or so, to allow the flavors time to marry. At this point, the soup can be refrigerated and reheated the following day (the soup will actually taste better the next day).

▸ When ready to serve, stir in the fresh lemon juice and taste for salt.

MIXED VEGETABLE WAT (SPICY STEW)

A *wat* is a spicy Ethiopian stew made with *berbere*, an Ethiopian spice blend, heavy on the hot pepper. Leave it out or be judicious with it unless you know your family likes it spicy.

The richly seasoned *Niter Kebbeh* oil adds an amazing flavor to this dish, so don't be tempted to skip it. ("These are the best vegetables I've ever had!" my son once exclaimed.)

Serve the mixed vegetable wat with Ethiopian Injera Bread (page 225) and eat it in the traditional Ethiopian manner, by tearing off pieces of the bread and scooping up bites of the spicy stew.

Makes 4 servings

1/2 recipe (scant 1/4 cup) Niter Kebbeh
   (page 101)
1 onion, minced
1 garlic clove, minced
1/2 a red bell pepper, chopped
1 tablespoon tomato paste
2 large carrots, cut into 1/2-inch slices
2 cups peeled new potatoes, cut into
   3/4-inch cubes
A pinch of berbere (or cayenne)
2 cups mixed vegetables (cauliflower or
   broccoli florets, fresh green beans,
   large slices of zucchini, and so on)
1 teaspoon salt (or to taste)
Black pepper
1 cup frozen peas

▶ Heat the Niter Kebbeh in a large saucepan over medium heat. Sauté the onion until soft, about 5 minutes. Add the garlic and bell pepper and sauté an additional minute. Add the tomato

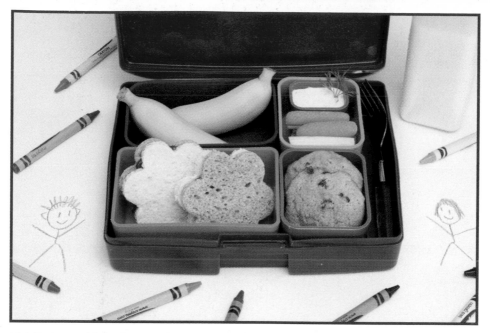

Nut Butter and Jelly Cutouts (page 133), baby bananas, and carrot and celery sticks with Easy Ranch Dip (page 106), with Back-to-School Chocolate Chip Cookies (page 232), and fortified soymilk.

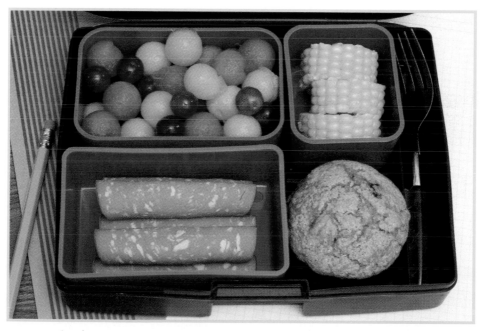

Vegan Deli Slice Roll-Ups (page 139), Corn Tires (page 9), grapes and melon balls, and Pumpkin Carob Chip Muffin (page 214).

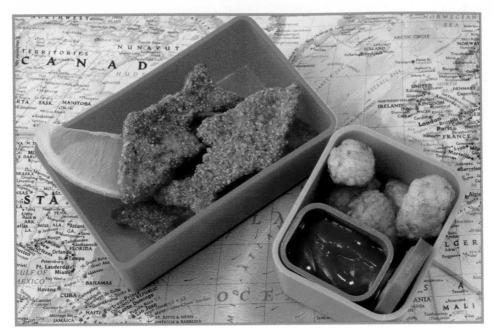

Tofu Fish Sticks (page 182), Tater Tots (page 22), and ketchup.

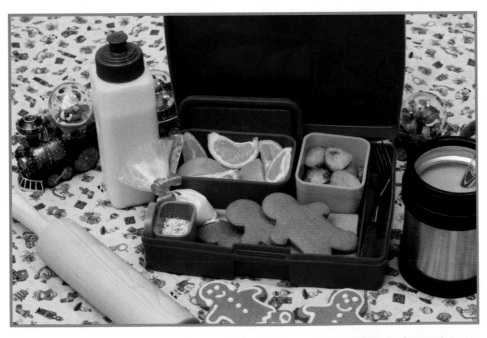

Golden Chestnut Soup (page 117), Best Brussels Sprouts (page 191), a clementine, soy nog (page 58), and Gingerbread Vegans with icing and sprinkles (page 238).

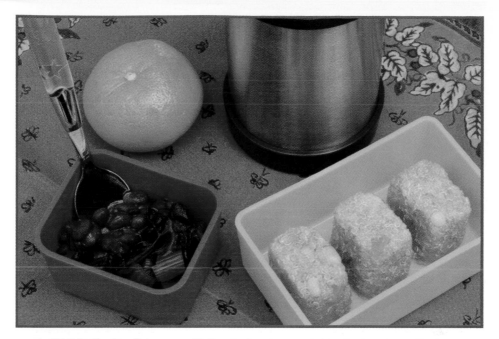

Quinoa Amaranth Timbales (page 169), Slow Cooker Black Beans (page 204), steamed swiss chard, and a tangerine.

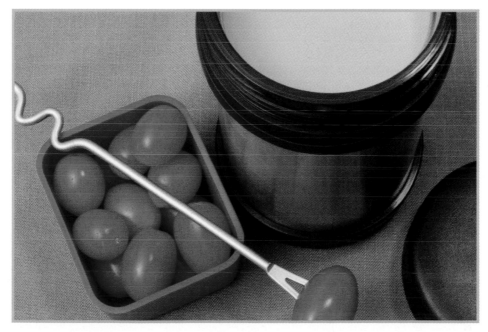

Lunch Box Fondue (page 72) with cherry tomatoes.

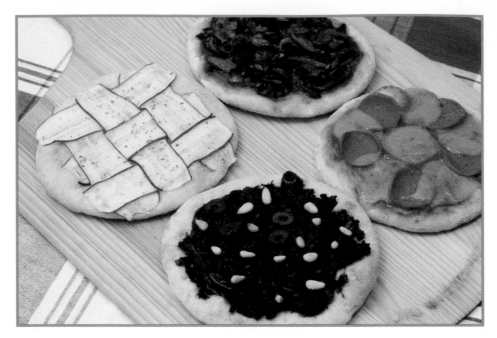

Mini Vegan Pizzas (clockwise from left): Zucchini Lattice (page 161), Mixed Mushroom (page 163), Polka-Dot Pepperoni (page 163), and Kale Kalamata (page 162).

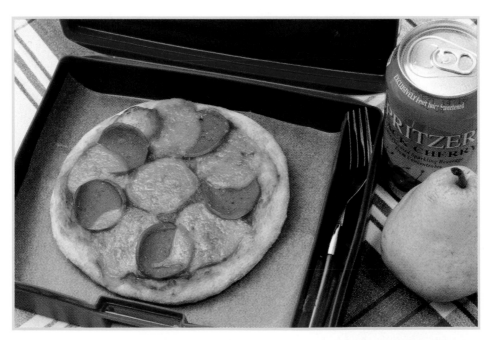

Polka-Dot Pepperoni Mini Pizza with a pear and a fruit-sweetened soda (page 163).

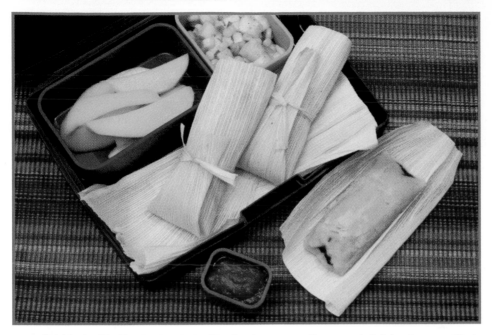

Black Bean Tamales (page 146), salsa, fresh mango slices, and Calabacita con Elote (page 193).

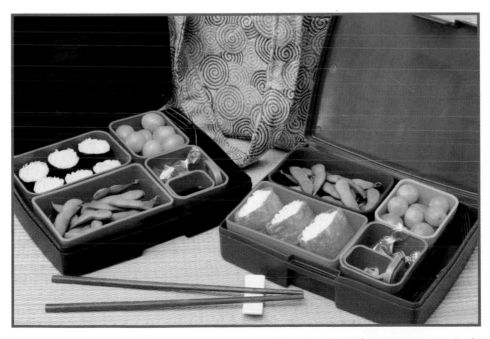

Sushi Rolls (page 178), Edamame, grapes, Botan Rice Candy, and soy sauce; Inari Sushi (page 158), Edamame, green grapes, Botan Rice Candy, and pickled ginger.

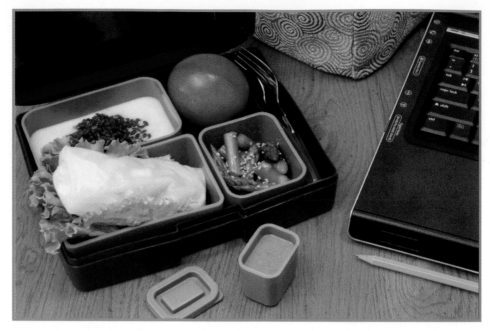

Tofu Apple Spring Roll (page 87) with Quick Peanut Sauce (page 108), Ted's Asian Asparagus (page 205), Black Rice Pudding (page 247), and a nectarine.

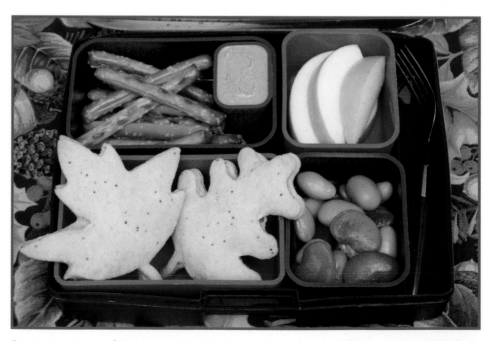

Savory Autumn Leaf Pies (page 172), pretzel sticks with peanut butter, green apple slices, and mixed lima and cannellini beans.

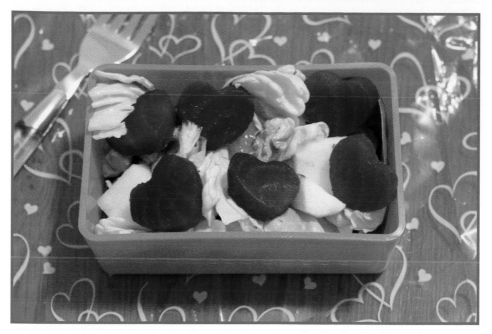

Valentine's Day Heart Beet Salad (page 99).

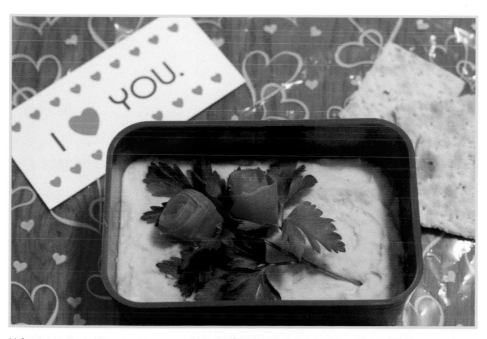

Valentine's Day Tomato Roses on a Bed of Cannellini Bean Puree (page 110).

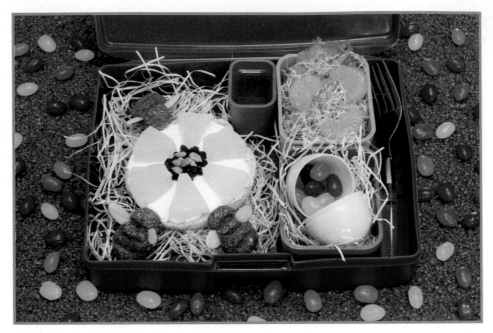

Sunflower Sandwich (page 137) surrounded by Honeybee No-Bakes (page 241), Sprout Salad with Mandarin Orange Dressing (page 103), and a plastic egg filled with vegan jelly beans.

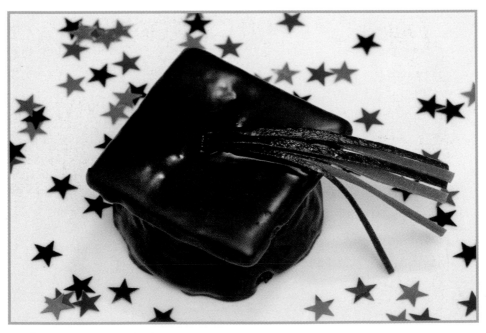

Graduation Hat (page 251).

paste, carrots, potatoes, berbere, and 1 cup water. Bring to a boil and lower the heat. Simmer, partially covered, for 10 minutes, then add the mixed vegetables and cook for another 10 minutes, or until all the vegetables are tender. Add the salt, pepper to taste, and frozen peas. Cover and cook until the peas are tender, about 2 minutes.

▶ Serve directly on top of injera bread, tearing off pieces of the bread to scoop up the stew, or serve in a bowl on the side. Pack for lunch in a sealed container at room temperature or in a preheated insulated food jar, with pieces of injera bread packed separately to scoop up the wat at lunchtime.

VARIATION: Instead of peas, top the stew with four 1-inch wedges of fresh green cabbage. Simmer until the cabbage is tender.

ROASTED TOMATO BASIL SOUP

Here it is—the recipe that transformed my son into a tomato lover! Tomato soup is all warmth and comfort on a cold winter day, and this one is as vibrant, creamy, and flavorful as it gets. I make and freeze large batches of this soup in the summertime when our tomato plants are overflowing with fruit. But you can make it anytime: roasting punches up the flavor of even grocery store tomatoes.

Makes 4 servings

6–6½ pounds plum tomatoes, cut in half lengthwise (about 35)

¼ cup plus 1 tablespoon extra virgin olive oil

1 tablespoon kosher salt

½ a medium onion, chopped

1 large garlic clove, minced

1 teaspoon red pepper flakes

2 cups fresh whole basil leaves
(one 2-ounce bag)
½ teaspoon dried thyme

- ▸ Preheat the oven to 400°F.
- ▸ Arrange the cut tomatoes on a large (10 x 16-inch) baking sheet. Drizzle the tomatoes with ¼ cup olive oil and sprinkle with salt. Toss with your hands until the tomatoes are evenly coated with oil, then arrange them cut side up; they should fill the pan completely. Place in oven and roast the tomatoes for 50 minutes. Remove pan from the oven and set aside.
- ▸ Warm the rest of the olive oil in a large saucepan over medium heat. Add the onion and sauté until soft and slightly golden, about 10 minutes. Add garlic and pepper flakes and sauté for one more minute. Carefully pour in all the tomatoes and their juices. Add the basil, thyme, and 1 cup water (you may need to add an extra cup if the tomatoes are on the dry side). Simmer for 15 minutes. Remove from heat and allow to cool slightly.
- ▸ Blend the soup in batches in the blender, pouring finished soup into a clean saucepan or soup tureen (you may wish to strain the soup as you do this to remove any remaining skin or seeds, depending on the strength of your blender).
- ▸ Serve piping hot, with crackers or chunks of store-bought artisan-style bread.

ROASTED VEGETABLE BROTH

This lovely golden broth adds flavor to soups, stews, and sauces and is so much better than anything you can buy in a box. Roasting brings out the flavor of the vegetables.

Makes about
10 cups

2 large onions, peeled and quartered

2 leeks, roots and dark green portions cut
away, halved lengthwise and rinsed well

3 large carrots, peeled and cut into
$3/4$-inch pieces

4 celery stalks, cut into $3/4$-inch pieces

1 fennel bulb, end and stalks removed,
cut into sixths

$1/2$ a red bell pepper, seeded and
cut into strips

1 tablespoon extra virgin olive oil

6 large garlic cloves, peeled and crushed
slightly

8 sprigs fresh parsley

6 sprigs fresh thyme or $1/2$ teaspoon
dried thyme

1 bay leaf

6 whole black peppercorns

2 tablespoons nutritional yeast flakes

$3/4$ teaspoon salt

▸ Preheat the oven to 450°F. Place the onions, leeks, carrots, celery, fennel, and red bell pepper in a 9 x 13-inch baking dish and toss with the olive oil. Roast for 30 minutes, stirring once halfway through.

- Put the vegetables into a large stockpot with 11 cups of water. Add the garlic, herbs, nutritional yeast, and salt. Bring to a boil, then lower the heat and simmer, lid slightly ajar, for 30 to 60 minutes. Strain.
- The stock can be used right away, refrigerated for up to a week, or frozen in serving-size portions for several months.

SNEAKY MOMMA'S BLACK BEAN SOUP

Creamy, pureed soups can hide a number of nutritious vegetables. My zucchini-, onion- and pepper-hating son calls this "the best soup I ever ate!"

Makes 3½ cups

1 tablespoon extra virgin olive oil

¼ onion, chopped

¼ red bell pepper, chopped

1 garlic clove, minced

1 teaspoon ground cumin

1 medium zucchini, peeled and chopped

1 tomato, peeled, seeded, and chopped (or one canned tomato, drained and chopped)

2 (15-ounce) cans black beans, or about 3½ cups cooked black beans, drained and rinsed

½ teaspoon oregano

¾ teaspoon salt (or to taste)

Freshly ground black pepper

- Heat the olive oil in a saucepan over medium-high heat. Add the onion and bell pepper and cook, stirring frequently, until the onion is softened and beginning to brown, about 4 minutes. Add the garlic and cumin. Stir briefly, about 30 seconds, then add the zucchini, tomato, and 1½ cups water. Bring to a boil, then turn heat to low and simmer, covered, until the zucchini is tender, about 5 minutes.

▶ Measure out 1 cup of the black beans and set them aside. Put the rest of the beans and the oregano into the saucepan.

▶ Transfer the soup to a blender, in batches if necessary, and puree until thick, smooth, and creamy. Pour soup into a clean saucepan and return to the stove on medium-low heat.

▶ Add the whole beans and the salt. Cook, stirring, until warmed through. Add a bit more water if the soup is too thick for your taste. Taste for salt, season with pepper to taste, and serve.

THOUGHTS ON THERMOSES

Once when I was in middle school, my mom packed me an insulated food jar (also known as a Thermos) filled with pasta for lunch. I was mortified. I positively burned with embarrassment at the thought of eating food from a food jar. Cool kids did *not* pack a warm lunch.

Skip ahead a few years to my son's first grade classroom and hey, the Thermos is in! Everyone who is anyone has an insulated food jar to carry hot items for lunch. There are food jars covered with cartoon characters, pink food jars, multicolored food jars with folding sporks that fit inside the lids. We found our stainless steel wide-mouth Thermos at a local grocery store. It holds 10 ounces—the perfect size for a kid-size serving of soup, beans, or fondue.

Always preheat your insulated food jar by filling it with boiling water, covering it with the lid, and setting it aside for 10 minutes while you heat up your soup or stew. Drain and dry with a clean towel before filling.

SPLIT PEA ALECHA (STEW)

If you are making Split Pea Alecha in advance, be aware that the stew will thicken considerably as it cools. Simply add a couple tablespoons of water when reheating. The stew should not be too thin—it should remain thick enough to scoop up with Ethiopian Injera Bread (page 225).

Makes 4 servings

----
1 1/2 cups dried split peas, rinsed and drained
1/4 teaspoon turmeric
1/2 recipe (scant 1/4 cup) Niter Kebbeh
   (page 101)
1 small onion, diced
3/4 teaspoon salt (or to taste)

▸ In a large saucepan, combine the split peas with 5 cups water and sprinkle with the turmeric. Bring to a boil and lower the heat. Simmer, partially covered, until the liquid has thickened and the split peas have lost their shape, about 60 to 70 minutes. Stir the split peas frequently during the last 20 minutes of cooking to keep them from sticking to the bottom of the pan.

▸ Meanwhile, heat the Niter Kebbeh in a small skillet over medium heat. When hot, add the onion and sauté, stirring frequently, until the onion is completely soft, about 10 minutes. When the split peas are done, add in the onion mixture and the salt and stir well to combine.

▸ Serve directly on top of the Ethiopian Injera Bread, tearing off pieces of the bread to scoop up the stew. Pack for lunch in a preheated insulated food jar, with pieces of injera bread packed separately to scoop up the alecha at lunchtime.

SANDWICHES

"OKAY, I'VE GOT TWO PIECES OF BREAD. NOW WHAT?"

If you're new to veganism, it may seem hard to imagine sandwiches without meat, eggs, or cheese. Here's a small sampling of ideas for vegan sandwich fillings to help get you started!

- nut butter with jam or fruit spread
- vegan cream cheese, strawberry jam, and cashews
- mashed beans and chopped pickle
- avocado, sprouts, lettuce, and tomato
- mixed green salad with salad dressing
- baked or smoked tofu
- Chickpea Salad (see page 94)
- vegan pâté (available at health food stores)
- cashew butter and banana

continues

- leftover Wheat Gluten Pot Roast and Gravy (see page 184) with ketchup
- sliced tofu hot dog with ketchup and mustard
- Veggie Tea Sandwiches (see page 141)
- peanut butter with grated carrot and mung bean sprouts
- Grilled Pepperoni Sandwich (see page 130)
- vegan deli slices with Vegenaise, lettuce, and tomato
- almond butter and chopped dates or a mashed date-coconut roll
- Imitation vegan tuna mixed with Vegenaise, black pepper, chopped celery, onion, and pickle
- vegan cheese (see "Gettin' Cheesy," page 131)
- Tofurky with vegan cream cheese and cranberry sauce
- sunflower seed butter with raisins and Sneaky Cinnamon-Sugar (page 29)
- Veggie Burger (see page 140)
- roasted red peppers, marinated artichoke hearts, and black olive tapenade
- Lentil-Rice Balls (page 159) mashed with tomato sauce or ketchup
- Easy Hummus (see page 105) with cucumber slices and black olives
- baba ganoush (eggplant dip) with grilled zucchini
- falafel balls with hummus, tahini (sesame seed butter), and lettuce
- vegan "chicken" patties with Vegenaise and mustard
- mixed grilled zucchini, eggplant, and onion slices
- vegan cream cheese mixed with canned crushed pineapple
- almond butter and apple slices
- refried beans mixed with salsa

- mixed roasted vegetables topped with pesto or basil puree
- fried tempeh
- peanut butter and kiwi fruit
- margarine with spicy pumpkin, apple, or pear butter
- grilled portobello mushroom with caramelized onions and a drizzle of balsamic vinegar
- vegan bacon with Vegenaise, lettuce, and Oven-Dried Tomatoes (page 200)
- scrambled tofu
- vegan coleslaw and toasted cashews
- dried figs, soaked overnight to soften, then mashed with ground hazelnuts or hazelnut butter
- soynut butter with jam or fruit spread
- golden-fried tofu with Quick Peanut Sauce (page 108) and baby spinach
- a thin layer of Vegemite or Marmite (yeast extract) topped with avocado and tomato
- baked beans
- herb and chive vegan cream cheese with sprouts, red onion, lettuce, and tomato
- a slice of leftover "meatloaf" with ketchup or chutney (visit my "Magical Loaf Studio" to create your very own loaf: www.veganlunchbox.com/loaf_studio.html)
- peanut butter and vegan chocolate or carob chips

P.S. To keep your sandwiches from becoming soggy, pack the filling ingredients separately and assemble the sandwich just before eating. If using nut butters, vegan cream cheese, or margarine, spreading some on both sides of the bread will also help prevent the sogs.

GRILLED PEPPERONI SANDWICH

An interesting and very easy variation on pizza!

This sandwich is lightly toasted in a skillet before packing. But since it won't still be hot at lunchtime, what's the point? Well, we still enjoy the crispy crunch of the toasted bread, and the once-melted cheese helps hold the sandwich together.

Makes 1 sandwich

---

2 slices of sandwich bread
9 slices of vegan pepperoni
2 slices of vegan mozzarella-style cheese
    (see "Gettin' Cheesy," page 131)
Extra virgin olive oil
Sneaky Momma's Tomato Sauce (page 109)
    or store-bought pizza sauce

▸ Lay one slice of vegan cheese on a slice of bread, then evenly distribute the vegan pepperoni slices over the cheese. Top the pepperoni with the other slice of cheese, then cover with the other slice of bread.

▸ Heat a drizzle of olive oil in a small skillet and grill the sandwich until the bread is brown and crisp on the outside.

▸ Cut the sandwich in half and wrap in a paper towel or foil. Pack the sandwich in a sealed lunch container along with a small container of tomato sauce for dipping.

GETTIN' CHEESY

Be sure to read labels when looking for vegan cheese; most "nondairy" cheeses still contain dairy in the form of casein, so watch out. Several brands of vegan block cheeses and slices are available in the refrigerated section of health food and grocery stores.

Common brands include Tofutti and VeganRella. These cheeses are usually made from soy and can be used in most recipes that call for regular cheese.

As I write this, Tofutti slices are the only vegan cheeses available in our local area. They're tasty, and our son enjoys them as an occasional treat. Unfortunately, they contain hydrogenated oil, so we try to go easy on them. Vegan Gourmet by Follow Your Heart (www.followyourheart .com) is considered by many to be the best vegan cheese in the states, but it is not currently widely available. I have also heard reports of good vegan cheeses in other parts of the world—Cheezly in the United Kingdom and Scheese in Scotland are two. Shop around and try out the different brands available in your area and see what you like.

If you're feeling adventurous and oh-so-clever, you can try making your own vegan block cheeses from scratch. I like to make vegan "cheese sticks" for lunches, using some of the block cheese recipes found in vegan cookbooks such as *Dairy-Free and Delicious* and *The Ultimate Uncheese Cookbook* (see Recommended Resources on page 261). I pour the warm "cheese" mixture into an oiled ice stick tray to cool, forming sticks that can be eaten as a finger food.

HAZELNUT BANANA SANDWICH BITES

Hazelnut butter makes an interesting alternative to peanut butter in these little sandwiches. It has a rich, sweet flavor that pairs nicely with bananas or chocolate.

Kids love it when I serve these easy bites using party toothpicks topped with umbrellas or paper fruit.

> 2 or 3 sandwich
> bites make a
> good serving

Special equipment you will need:
A small circular cookie cutter
    (about 1 1/2 inches across)

Hazelnut butter
A banana, sliced into rounds
Whole-grain sandwich bread

▸ Use a small circular cookie cutter to cut out circles of bread that are just a bit bigger than a slice of banana. Spread the bread rounds with hazelnut butter and sandwich a banana slice in the middle.

▸ Poke a fun party toothpick through the middle of each sandwich to hold the bite-sized sandwiches together (make sure any sharp ends are trimmed off before serving them to a younger child).

VARIATION: Chocolate Hazelnut Banana Bites: Add a bit of vegan chocolate syrup to the hazelnut butter.

NUT BUTTER AND JELLY CUTOUTS

When cutting out sandwiches with cookie cutters, cut the bread first before spreading on the nut butter and jam; the bread will hold its shape better and you won't waste any filling. If you're a frugal mom, as I am, you can save the leftover bread and crusts and make them into croutons or breadcrumbs to use in other recipes.

Also, when making any nut butter and jelly sandwich to go, always spread a thin layer of nut butter on both inner sides of the sandwich to keep the jam from soaking into the bread and becoming soggy in the lunch box.

Makes 1 serving

Special equipment you will need:
Cookie cutters

2 slices of sandwich bread
All-natural peanut butter or other nut butter
Fruit-sweetened jam

▸ Use cookie cutters to cut shapes out of the bread one at a time, then spread a thin layer of nut butter on both slices of bread. Make sure to use corresponding sides of the bread so the cutout shapes will line up when placed together (hey, if you're making these at 6 a.m., this could be a helpful reminder). Spread a thin layer of jam on one slice and press the slices together, crimping with your fingers along any pointed edges to help the sandwich stay together.

VARIATION: Try using one slice of white bread and one slice of wheat for a two-tone sandwich.

PEANUT BUTTER AND JELLY POP HEARTS

Here's a treat to make for your own little sweethearts, on Valentine's Day or any day. Heart-shaped pastry cutouts are filled with nut butter and jelly for a very different take on PB&J. These hearts can be eaten cold for lunch or warmed up in a toaster for breakfast.

Makes 10 (4-inch) Pop Hearts

Special equipment you will need:
A 4-inch heart-shaped cookie cutter

1 recipe Easy Piecrust (page 211)
10 tablespoons peanut or other nut butter
10 tablespoons jam, jelly, or fruit spread

▸ Preheat the oven to 400°F. Line a baking sheet with parchment paper, spray with nonstick spray, and set aside.

▸ Prepare a batch of Easy Piecrust, either the white or half whole wheat version. Roll the piecrust out on a floured surface and cut it into heart shapes using a 4-inch cookie cutter.

▸ Place one heart on the prepared baking sheet. Dab a spoonful of nut butter into the center of the heart and top with a spoonful of your favorite fruit spread or jam. Spread out the butter and jam using the back of a spoon, leaving a half inch of space all around the edges. Brush the edges with cold water and top with another heart. Press the edges together and crimp all around with a fork.

▸ Bake for 20 minutes, or until lightly browned.

VARIATION: When the Pop Hearts are cool, you can decorate them with any favorite icing or frosting (powdered sugar mixed with juice or nondairy milk makes an easy, quick icing). I like to use a pastry bag fitted with a small round tip to write little messages such as "Be Mine" on the tops of my Pop Hearts, rather like the candy hearts you see on Valentine's Day. Frosted Pop Hearts can be warmed up while lying flat in a toaster oven or oven, but I fear the frosting would make a mess in a regular toaster.

PITA SANDWICH WITH FLAXY HUMMUS

Hummus, a creamy bean spread traditionally made with chickpeas (also known as garbanzo beans), is a perennial vegetarian favorite. This recipe can even supply your children with their daily serving of healthy omega–3 fatty acids from ground flax.

Hummus is getting easier to find at most large grocery stores, health food stores, and delis. For this recipe, you can use your favorite home-made or store-bought hummus, or try the simple recipe on page 105.

This recipe can easily be doubled or tripled to suit your needs.

Makes 1 serving

½ a piece of white or whole wheat pita bread

3 tablespoons Easy Hummus (page 105) or your favorite homemade or store-bought hummus

1 teaspoon ground flaxseed

Optional additions:
Sprouts
Lettuce or baby spinach
Oven-Dried Tomatoes (page 200)
Black or Kalamata olives

▸ Place the hummus into a small bowl and stir in the ground flaxseed until well blended. Use a butter knife to fill the pita bread with an even layer of hummus.

▸ You can cut the filled pita into wedges to serve as an easy finger food, or fill the pita with any or all of the optional additions for a sandwich.

SCARY SPIDER SANDWICHES

Circular chocolate graham crackers make up the bodies of these spooky spiders. Crisp chow mein noodles make fine squiggly, squirmy spider legs, or use pretzels for longer, straight ones.

Spicy pumpkin butter or apple butter makes a fine fall sandwich filling when mixed with peanut butter.

Makes 4 spiders (1 serving)	8 Chocolate Graham Crackers (page 66), shaped as 2-inch circles
	2 tablespoons natural peanut butter
	2 teaspoons store-bought pumpkin butter or apple butter
	Chow mein noodles or small pretzel sticks
	Pine nuts or raisins

▸ Prepare the graham crackers the day before.

▸ In the morning, mix the peanut butter with the pumpkin or apple butter in a small bowl. Spread a thick layer of the peanut butter mixture on each graham cracker. Press eight chow mein noodles or pretzel sticks along the edges of half of the graham crackers to make spider legs, and top with the other graham crackers. Dab a bit of the peanut butter mixture onto the pine nuts or raisins and press them onto the tops of the graham crackers to make eyes.

▸ To pack, tear white paper towels into strips and crunch them up to make a bed of "mummy wrap." Rest the spiders gently on top and cover with another paper towel so they don't get jostled in the lunch box.

SUNFLOWER SANDWICH

These are as tasty as they are adorable! The flavors of vegan cream cheese and pineapple go so well together.

Makes 1 serving

$\frac{1}{2}$ an English muffin (or any round-shaped bread or bun)

Vegan cream cheese or nut butter

1 dried pineapple ring

Currants

Toasted, unsalted sunflower seeds

▸ Spread the English muffin with a generous layer of vegan cream cheese or nut butter.

▸ Cut the dried pineapple ring into 6 to 8 wedges. Arrange the pineapple wedges around the perimeter of the English muffin to resemble the petals of a flower.

▸ Place a small heap of currants mixed with sunflower seeds in the middle of the English muffin to resemble the center of a sunflower.

TORTILLA ROLL-UPS

A tortilla rolled up with refried beans makes a quick, easy meal and has become one of our lunch-in-a-hurry standbys. Older children can easily put this lunch together themselves.

Makes 1 serving

1 whole wheat, white, or spelt tortilla
2–3 tablespoons Refried Black Beans
    (page 203, or use any canned
    refried beans)
½ teaspoon ground cumin (optional)

▸ Lay the tortilla out on a cutting board. Using a small spatula, spread a thin layer of beans across the surface of the tortilla. Sprinkle with cumin, if using.

▸ Starting at the base, roll the tortilla up tightly. Lay the tortilla seam side down, and cut into 2-inch pieces using a serrated knife.

▸ Pack along with a small container of salsa for dipping, if you like.

VEGAN DELI SLICE ROLL-UPS

Even young kids can make these for themselves with just a bit of help getting the roll started.

> **3 to 5 roll-ups make a good serving**

1 package vegan deli slices (ham, turkey, bologna, and so on)

Vegan cream cheese

▸ Working with one deli slice at a time, pat the deli slice dry with a kitchen towel. Using a butter knife, spread one side of the deli slice with vegan cream cheese.

▸ Roll the slice up (the inner edge of the roll may tear a bit when you start rolling, so be gentle). Press gently to seal, and stack them in the lunch container.

VARIATION: Zucchini Roll-Ups: Place a small raw baby zucchini at the edge of the cream cheese–covered deli slice and roll it up.

VEGGIE BURGER

There are dozens of vegan veggie burgers on the market today. You can find them in the freezer, refrigerator, or even the canned food section of almost any grocery or health food store. We especially like the dried veggie burger mixes that you add water to and form into patties; these economical dried mixes can sometimes be found in bulk bins, saving money and packaging. Some veggie burgers taste quite a bit like meat; others taste more of brown rice, beans, mushrooms, or mixed veggies. Try them all and find out which ones you prefer.

Pan toasting the bun adds a nice flavor and keeps the bread from getting soggy in the lunch box.

Makes 1
veggie burger

1 vegan burger patty

1 slice of vegan cheese (optional)

1 hamburger bun

Extra virgin olive oil

Vegenaise, barbecue sauce, ketchup,
   or mustard (optional)

Lettuce, tomato, red onion, or other
   veggies (optional)

▸ Prepare the burger patty by frying it in a nonstick skillet with a drizzle of olive oil or cook according to package directions. Top with a slice of vegan cheese, if desired. Cover the pan to retain heat and cook until the cheese is warmed through.

▸ Meanwhile, heat a large nonstick or cast-iron skillet over medium heat. Add a drizzle of olive oil to the pan. Slice the bun in half and place pieces cut-side down in the pan. Sear the bun until it is toasted and warmed through, about 1 minute.

▸ Spread the bread with Vegenaise and/or ketchup and mustard if desired. Place the burger patty inside the bun topped with your assortment of fresh veggies (if you won't be eating the burger for a while, you may wish to pack the vegetables separately in a resealable plastic bag, then add them at mealtime). Wrap the sandwich in parchment paper and/or foil and pack in a sealed container.

VEGGIE TEA SANDWICHES

Tea sandwiches are so dainty and fun to eat. You might be surprised at how good radish sandwiches taste! Try making two or three varieties and alternating them in a row in a lunch container.

Save the crusts you cut away and pulse them in a food processor to make breadcrumbs for veggie burger patties. Breadcrumbs can be stored in the freezer.

---

4 bite-size
sandwiches equal
1 serving

Good-quality sandwich bread, including white,
wheat, light rye, or Pumpernickel,
crusts removed

Fillings of choice (see below)

▶ Use a bread knife to cut the bread into thin rectangles, triangles, or squares, or use sharp cookie cutters to cut the sandwiches into fun shapes. (Traditional tea sandwiches should be large enough to be eaten in two bites.) Spread two corresponding pieces of bread with a thin layer of margarine, Vegenaise, or cream cheese and fill with the vegetable of your choice.

Classic tea sandwich filling combinations include the following:

- radish slices with margarine
- peeled cucumber slices with vegan cream cheese and fresh dill
- peeled cucumber slices with margarine and fresh mint

- lightly blanched slim asparagus stalks with Vegenaise
- chopped celery and walnuts mixed with vegan cream cheese
- watercress or arugula with margarine

"EAT YOUR CRUSTS . . ."

Be careful serving these tea sandwiches—your son or daughter may ask for crustless bread from now on! If they do, here are some tried-and-true "mom-isms" to get crusts back in your kid's good graces:

"They're the most nutritious part!"

Did you know that this might actually be true? In 2002, German researchers found that the cancer-fighting antioxidant pronyllysine is concentrated in the crust of bread.

"They'll put hair on your chest!" Uh, and is that a good thing?

And a personal favorite from my own mom:

"They help you whistle!"

MAINS

ALOO SAMOSAS

These savory hand pies travel well and are simple to prepare. Traditional Indian *samosas* are deep-fried, but here they are baked. "I looove this filling," says James, between mouthfuls.

Makes 18 samosas

1 ½ pounds russet potatoes (about 3 medium), peeled and quartered

¾ cup frozen green peas

½ teaspoon ground cumin

½ teaspoon turmeric

¼ teaspoon cayenne (or to taste)

½ teaspoon kosher salt (or to taste)

Freshly ground black pepper

1 tablespoon finely minced fresh cilantro

One recipe Easy Piecrust (page 211)

Extra virgin olive oil

- ▸ Spray a nonstick muffin tin with nonstick spray and set aside. Have a small rolling pin and a small bowl of water ready.
- ▸ To make the filling, place the potatoes in a medium saucepan and cover with water. Bring to a boil, lower the heat, and simmer, partially covered, until the potatoes are tender. Meanwhile, cook the green peas according to package directions, drain, and set aside.
- ▸ Drain the potatoes. Add the cumin, turmeric, cayenne, salt, and pepper to taste, and mash the potatoes coarsely using a potato masher. Add the peas and cilantro and mix together. Set aside to cool.
- ▸ Make the piecrust according to the directions on page 211. Divide the dough into eighteen equal pieces, each roughly the size of a walnut.
- ▸ Working with one piece at a time on a lightly floured work surface, roll the dough into a ball, then use the rolling pin to roll the ball into a flat, 5-inch-wide circle. Sprinkle the work surface and rolling pin with flour as necessary to keep the dough from sticking.
- ▸ Place a heaping 1½ tablespoons of potato filling in the center of the circle. Dip a finger in the bowl of water and run it around the edges of the dough to moisten it. Bring all the edges of the dough up, folding and gathering them together over the filling. Pinch with your fingers to seal. Repeat with the remaining dough and filling, placing each finished samosa in a muffin cup. Spray or brush the finished samosas with olive oil.
- ▸ At this point, the samosas can be baked immediately or refrigerated, covered with plastic wrap, for several hours or overnight.
- ▸ When ready to bake, preheat the oven to 400°F. Bake for 25 minutes, until warmed through and golden brown on the bottom.

VARIATION: Gobi Samosas: Replace all or part of the potatoes with cooked cauliflower for delicious gobi samosas.

BEANS AND DOGS

This recipe can easily be doubled, tripled, or even quadrupled to feed a crowd of hungry children; we often bring this to our monthly vegetarian potlucks so the kids are sure to find a dish they enjoy.

Makes 2 servings

1 (16-ounce) can vegetarian baked beans
Two soy hot dogs

▸ Bring a medium saucepan filled with water to a boil. Pour off some of the boiling water into your insulated food jar, and set it aside for 10 minutes to preheat as you finish making the dish.

▸ Set the soy hot dogs in the saucepan, covered with the remaining boiling water. Cover the saucepan and set aside for 2 minutes (or cook according to package directions). Meanwhile, heat the baked beans in a small saucepan or in the microwave.

▸ When the hot dogs are done, drain and pat dry. Slice the hot dogs into bite-size pieces (if making this for very young children, be sure to cut the hot dogs in halves or quarters to avoid a choking hazard) and stir them into the warm beans.

▸ Drain the food jar and wipe dry, then fill with Beans and Dogs.

BLACK BEAN TAMALES

Tamales aren't difficult, but they may seem intimidating if you've never made them before. Visit a Mexican grocery store or the ethnic section of your supermarket to find bags of dried corn husks and *masa harina* (a special cornmeal used for making tortillas) and start out with this small batch.

Makes 12 tamales

4 ounces dried corn husks
2 cups instant masa harina
1 teaspoon baking powder
3/4 teaspoon kosher salt
1/2 cup nonhydrogenated shortening
About 1 1/8 cups warm "no-chicken" or
    vegetable broth, plus more as needed
2 cups Refried Black Beans (page 203,
    or use any canned vegan refried beans)
Salsa

▸ Start the dried corn husks soaking in a sink full of warm water about 15 minutes before you begin so they can soften (put a lid or plate over the husks to keep them submerged).

▸ In a small bowl, mix together the masa harina, baking powder, and salt. Set aside.

▸ Using a handheld beater or a stand mixer fitted with the paddle attachment, cream the shortening until it is light and fluffy, about 1 minute. Add the masa to the shortening, alternating with the broth, until a light, nonsticky dough is formed. Use only as much broth as needed. Continue beating for 1 minute more.

▸ To shape the tamales, pat a large corn husk dry and lay it out with the tapered end facing you. Scoop out a 2-inch round ball of masa, and spread it into a 4-inch square in the middle of the husk about 3/4 of an inch down from the top of the husk.

- Spread 1½ tablespoons of refried beans down the center of the masa dough. Pick up the sides of the corn husk and fold them in, closing up the refried beans in masa. Fold up the tapered section of the husk to form the sealed bottom of the tamale (the top remains open). Tie up the tamale loosely using kitchen twine or a strip of corn husk.
- Set all the tamales upright on their folded bottoms in a large steamer basket with a bit of room between them for the steam to circulate. Steam over boiling water for 40 to 45 minutes, until the tamale dough pulls away easily from the corn husk.
- Serve tamales with salsa for dipping.
- Tamales refrigerate and freeze well. Reheat by steaming them for a few minutes or popping them in the microwave.

BROCCOLI CALZONES

These tasty "pizza pockets" are made the night before and then refrigerated until the morning. Calzones are a wonderful, kid-friendly food, a kind of stuffed "mini pizza."

Makes 8 calzones

One recipe Easy Whole-Grain Pizza Dough
    (page 224)
4 to 5 cups broccoli, washed and cut into
    bite-size pieces
³/₄ pound firm tofu, drained and crumbled
2 tablespoons freshly squeezed lemon juice
³/₄ teaspoon dried basil
1 teaspoon salt
¹/₈ teaspoon garlic powder
Extra virgin olive oil
Sneaky Momma's Tomato Sauce (page 109)
    or store-bought tomato sauce

- Make the pizza dough, then cut it into eight equal pieces. Shape dough into smooth balls and place them on a well-floured surface about 2 inches apart. Cover with plastic wrap and let the dough rise for 45 minutes.

- Line two baking sheets with parchment paper and dust with cornmeal. Set aside.

- Meanwhile, steam the broccoli in a steamer basket until tender when pierced with a knife, about 10 minutes. Allow to cool slightly, then put the broccoli on a cutting board and chop it into bite-size pieces. Place in a large mixing bowl and set aside.

- To make the tofu "ricotta," place tofu, lemon juice, basil, salt, and garlic powder in the bowl of a food processor fitted with the S blade. Process until the mixture has a fine, grainy texture like ricotta cheese. Fold the "ricotta" into the broccoli and mix together gently.

- On a lightly floured surface, roll a dough ball into a 7-inch-wide circle. Place about $\frac{1}{2}$ cup of filling just off the center of the circle. Lightly moisten the edges of the dough (it helps to have a glass of water handy to dip your fingers into) and fold the edges together. Press and roll the edge up slightly to seal.

- Place four calzones on each baking sheet and brush each lightly with olive oil. Cover well with plastic wrap and refrigerate the calzones overnight.

- In the morning, take the calzones out of the refrigerator and preheat the oven to 425°F. Bake for 20 to 25 minutes, until golden and warmed through. Let cool for 5 to 10 minutes, then wrap in clean parchment or foil. Pack with a small container of tomato sauce to dip or drizzle over the calzone.

CHILI CON "CARNE"

This chili uses inexpensive dried beans rather than canned and spends the day bubbling away in the slow cooker. Start it in the morning, and it will be ready in time for a delicious dinner when you get home from work.

The "carne" in this recipe is textured vegetable protein (TVP). TVP is made from defatted soy flour and has a chewy, meaty flavor and texture; it comes dried in the bulk bins at most natural food stores.

Makes 6 servings

1/2 cup dried black beans

1/2 cup dried pinto beans

1/2 cup dried navy beans

1 tablespoon extra virgin olive oil

1 onion, finely chopped

1/2 a green or red bell pepper, chopped

1 garlic clove, minced

1 teaspoon ground cumin

1 1/2 teaspoons paprika

1/2 teaspoon dried thyme

1/2 teaspoon dried sage

1 teaspoon dried oregano

A pinch of cayenne

1/2 cup uncooked lentils (black, brown, or crimson are all fine here, just not red)

1 cup dried, beef-style TVP granules

1 (6-ounce) can salt-free tomato paste

1 teaspoon salt (or to taste)

Freshly ground black pepper

▸ Combine the black beans, pinto beans, and navy beans in a mixing bowl. Rinse and drain the beans, then cover with a generous amount of water. Let the beans soak for several hours or overnight.

▸ Heat the olive oil in a skillet over medium-high heat. When the oil is hot, add the onion and bell pepper and sauté until the onion is translucent and soft, about 5 minutes. Add the garlic, cumin, paprika, thyme, sage, oregano, and cayenne and sauté, stirring constantly, for another 2 minutes, or until the garlic is soft and the spices are fragrant.

▸ Scrape the onion and spice mixture into the insert of a medium-size (2.5 to 3 quarts) slow cooker. Drain the dry beans and add them to the slow cooker along with the lentils, TVP, and tomato paste. Add 5 cups of boiling water and stir until everything is combined and there are no lumps of tomato paste.

▸ Cover the slow cooker and cook on high for 5 hours or on low for 8 hours, until the beans are tender. If you are around, give the chili a stir or two during the day to ensure even cooking.

▸ When the chili is done, stir in the salt and pepper to taste and serve hot.

VARIATION: "Picky Chili": I like to call our usual version of this recipe "James's Picky Chili." "I *love* chili," he says, "as long as it doesn't have any onions . . . or peppers . . . or chunks of tomato . . . or green stuff . . . and as long as it's not too spicy." Allllrighty, then. So I leave out the onions and peppers and my son is in Chili Heaven. Feel free to skip the onions yourself if you have an onion-hating child.

HEARTY CHILI SPUDS

Our local vegetarian group once hosted a "Baked Potato Bar" potluck: we supplied the baked potatoes and everyone brought their favorite toppings. There was vegan sour cream and bacon bits, of course, and broccoli and grated vegan cheese. But guess which topping arrived over and over? You guessed it—vegetarian chili! Lucky thing, too, because after we ran out of potatoes, we still had satisfying bowls of chili to eat.

Makes 6 servings

One recipe Chili Con "Carne" (page 149)

6 baking potatoes

▸ To bake potatoes, preheat the oven to 400°F. Scrub the potato skins to remove any surface dirt. Wrap each potato individually in a piece of foil or parchment paper so that the potatoes are completely enclosed.

▸ Place the potatoes directly on the rack in the oven and bake until they are soft and tender when poked with a finger, about 1 to 2 hours, depending on the size of the potato.

▸ If baking the potatoes a day ahead, store them, still wrapped, in the refrigerator. In the morning, warm them up briefly in the microwave.

▸ To pack, cut the baked potato almost in half with a sharp knife, then wrap the potato in clean foil or parchment. To eat, remove the wrap, open the spud, and spoon hot chili on top.

THE MULTITASKING OVEN

While you are baking these potatoes, wrap and bake some sweet potatoes or yams the same way. You can eat them hot from the oven with a dab of margarine, or use them to make Almond Buttered Sweet Potatoes (page 190).

COCONUT CARROT RICE PUDDING

The next time you cook brown rice, you'll want to make extra just so you can enjoy this wonderful dish, redolent of cinnamon, cardamom, and coconut.

Makes 6 servings

1 pound carrots, peeled and grated
   (3 cups grated)
1 (14-ounce) can light coconut milk
$\frac{1}{2}$ cup pure maple syrup
3 cups cooked brown basmati rice
$\frac{1}{2}$ teaspoon cinnamon
$\frac{1}{2}$ teaspoon ground cardamom
$\frac{1}{4}$ cup golden raisins
Ground flaxseed (optional)
Finely chopped unsalted pistachios (optional)

▸ Using the large holes of a hand grater, grate the carrot directly into a medium saucepan. Add the coconut milk and maple syrup and place on the stove over medium-high heat. Bring to a boil, then turn the heat to low and simmer, covered, stirring occasionally, until carrots are completely tender, about 15 minutes.

▸ Stir in the brown rice, cinnamon, cardamom, and raisins. Continue cooking, stirring occasionally, until the rice is heated through and the mixture has thickened slightly, 4 to 5 minutes.

▸ Remove from heat and allow to cool. When ready to serve or pack, place a serving of rice pudding into a dish or container. Stir in some ground flaxseed (up to one tablespoon per serving) and top with pistachios, if desired.

CORNISH PASTIES

Look for vegan "steak strips" in the freezer section, but be warned: if it's been several years since you tasted steak, you may find the first bite unsettling—they're very steaklike!

Makes 4 pasties

1 tablespoon extra virgin olive oil

½ (4-ounce) package frozen vegan steak strips (such as Morningstar Farms)

1 tablespoon nonhydrogenated margarine

1 medium turnip, peeled and cut in a ½-inch dice

1 medium-large potato, peeled and cut in a ½-inch dice

½ teaspoon Marmite, Vegemite, or other yeast extract

Freshly ground black pepper

1 recipe Easy Piecrust (page 211)

▸ Heat the olive oil in a nonstick skillet and cook the steak strips according to package instructions. Drain on paper towels. When cool, cut into ½-inch pieces and set aside.

▸ Heat the margarine in the skillet and add the turnip and potato. Turn the heat to low and cook, covered, until completely tender, about 15 minutes. Add the Marmite and pepper to taste and stir gently to combine, then add the steak pieces. Let cool completely while you prepare the piecrust.

▸ Line a baking sheet with parchment paper and spray with nonstick spray. Have a small bowl of water ready.

▸ To form the pasties, divide the piecrust into four equal pieces. Lightly flour a work surface and roll the dough out with a rolling pin to about ⅛ inch thick. Cut the pastry into a 7-inch-wide circle (use a small plate or saucer to help guide you). Cover half of the pastry with a quarter of the potato mixture, leaving about ½ inch uncovered around the edges.

▶ Dip your fingers in water and moisten the edges of the pastry, then fold over the dough. Use your fingers to pinch and curl up the edges all the way around. Repeat with the remaining pastry and filling. You may wish to use the pastry scraps to cut out decorative shapes and affix them to the pasty with a dab of water. Spray or brush the pasties with olive oil.

▶ At this point, the pasties may be refrigerated for several hours or overnight. When ready to bake, preheat the oven to 400°F. Bake the pasties for 25 minutes, until lightly browned and warmed through.

EASY PASTA AND BEANS

More of a creative technique to add to your repertoire than an exact recipe, Easy Pasta and Beans can be made in a flash with any favorite pasta shape, bean, pea, or veggie. It's always a kid pleaser, and the possibilities are endless!

Makes 3 servings

4 ounces pasta shapes (spirals, bows, macaroni, shells, and so on)

1 tablespoon extra virgin olive oil

1 small onion, diced, and/or 1 garlic clove, minced

1½ cups frozen lima beans or frozen shelled edamame or canned beans (drained and rinsed) or frozen peas

2 tablespoons minced fresh parsley

Salt

Freshly ground black or white pepper

▸ Bring a large saucepan of lightly salted water to boil over high heat. If using frozen lima beans or edamame, add the beans to the pot. Boil limas until tender (about 12 minutes), edamame until warmed through (about 5 minutes). Scoop them out and set them aside.

▸ Add the pasta to the boiling water and cook until tender (check package for cooking time).

▸ Meanwhile, heat the olive oil in a large skillet or sauté pan. Add the onion and/or garlic, and sauté, stirring frequently, until soft, about 5 to 10 minutes. Add ¼ cup water and your bean of choice, either the cooked limas, edamame, canned beans, or frozen peas. Simmer gently until heated through, and set aside.

▸ When the pasta is done, drain it in a colander and add it to the bean or pea mixture. Add the fresh parsley and an extra drizzle of olive oil, if desired, and toss to combine. Season with salt and pepper to taste.

VARIATIONS:

- Add a teaspoon of minced fresh rosemary to the onion when using lima beans.
- Add other mixed frozen veggies along with the frozen peas.
- Sauté garlic in sesame oil when using edamame and season with a dash of soy sauce and a sprinkle of toasted sesame seeds.
- Add some canned, chopped tomatoes and ½ teaspoon oregano to the onion and/or garlic when using canned white beans for pasta e fagioli.

"EAT YOUR OATMEAL" PANCAKES

A great new way to get kids to eat their oatmeal! These pancakes are wheat- and oil-free, and contain heart-healthy omega–3 fatty acids from flax. The leftover pancakes taste great cold and make a tasty snack either plain, rolled up with jam, or dipped in syrup. They can easily be made a day in advance and refrigerated.

Keep in mind that oats do not contain the same gluten that wheat does, so these pancakes may be more delicate than what you are used to. Make sure your griddle is well heated and oiled so the pancakes don't stick and make them small until you get the hang of it.

Makes about 20 small pancakes

---

1 3/4 cups oat flour

1/4 teaspoon kosher salt

1/4 teaspoon cinnamon

3 tablespoons ground flaxseed

2 cups plain, unsweetened soymilk, plus more as needed (don't substitute rice milk; soy really does work best here)

1 tablespoon applesauce

1 tablespoon maple syrup (or another tablespoon of applesauce)

2 teaspoons baking powder

▸ Whisk together the oat flour, salt, and cinnamon in a mixing bowl. Set aside.
▸ Put the ground flaxseed into a blender with the soymilk, applesauce, and maple syrup. Blend together for 1 minute. Pour the liquid into the dry ingredients and whisk well until smooth. Set the batter aside for about 10 minutes while you preheat a nonstick or well-seasoned cast-iron griddle. The mixture will thicken as it sits.

- When the griddle is hot, stir the baking powder into the batter. Add a few tablespoons of water to thin the mixture to pancake batter consistency.
- Lightly oil your griddle or spray it with nonstick spray if necessary. When the griddle is nice and hot, pour out a small amount of batter, about 3 inches in diameter, and cook until the bottom is nicely browned and the sides are dry. Insert a spatula underneath the pancake and flip. Cook until this side is also browned and the center springs back gently to the touch.
- Serve these pancakes with fruit, nut butter, applesauce (my favorite is apple blackberry sauce), and/or maple syrup.

VARIATION: "Eat Your Oatmeal" Waffles: This batter also makes fantastic waffles. Follow recipe above but pour the batter into a preheated nonstick waffle iron that has been sprayed with nonstick spray. How many waffles and the cooking time will depend on your waffle iron. My iron makes two large squares (four waffles each) at 8 minutes each.

- For a great lunch, spread some peanut or almond butter between two waffles and cut the waffles into strips. Pack with a small container of maple syrup or some applesauce for dipping.

INARI SUSHI

Seasoned inari sushi pouches are available in cans at Asian markets. They are golden pockets made from fried tofu that are gently opened and stuffed with rice. They have a mild taste and make a great introduction to sushi for those who haven't tried it yet.

Makes 16 pouches

½ recipe prepared sushi rice (1 cup dry rice)

1 (10-ounce) can inari pouches (also called *inari zushi no moto*)

Optional toppings:
sesame seeds, pickled ginger, or grated carrot

▸ Prepare the sushi rice according to instructions beginning on page 178.

▸ Open the can of inari pouches and drain (you can save the liquid to moisten your fingers as you prepare the inari). Gently open one side of the inari pouch with your fingers or the tip of a sharp knife.

▸ Dip your fingers in the inari liquid or vinegared water (to keep the rice from sticking). Scoop up a large ball of rice and fill the inari pouch.

▸ Top with any of the optional toppings, or serve as is. Inari is traditionally not dipped in soy sauce, but you may do so if you like.

FRUGAL SUSHI MOMMA TIP

You may end up with one or two torn inari pouches that do not want to open (at least I always do). Don't throw them away! You can slice these into strips and use them as a filling in Sushi Rolls (page 178). Inari strips also go well with raw spinach and grated carrot in thick-rolled sushi (*futomaki-zushi*) or by themselves in narrow-rolled sushi (*hosomaki-zushi*).

LENTIL-RICE BALLS

If you cook up these savory Lentil-Rice Balls to serve with pasta and tomato sauce for dinner, the leftovers will make a fine, quickly assembled lunch the next day. Or you can prepare and store the shaped, uncooked balls in the refrigerator overnight and bake them in the morning especially for the lunch box. Pack the tomato sauce separately, so the balls don't get soggy.

Makes 22 balls, about 5 servings

$^1/_2$ cup brown rice, rinsed and drained

$^1/_2$ cup uncooked lentils, rinsed and drained (use green, brown, black, or crimson lentils, not red)

$^1/_2$ cup whole wheat flour

$^3/_4$ teaspoon baking powder

$^1/_2$ teaspoon salt (or to taste)

1 teaspoon Italian herb seasoning blend

$^1/_4$ teaspoon garlic granules

1 teaspoon cumin

Freshly ground black pepper

▸ Place the rice and lentils in a small saucepan and add 2 cups of water. Bring to a boil, lower the heat, and cover with a lid. Cook on low for 30 to 40 minutes, until rice and lentils are soft (or as one tester put it, "quite gooshy and easy to squish"). Remove from heat and drain the rice and lentils thoroughly in a fine mesh sieve to remove any excess water.

▸ Preheat the oven to 350°F. Line a baking sheet with parchment paper and spray with nonstick spray and set aside.

▸ When the rice and lentils are cool enough to touch, place them in a mixing bowl and add the flour, baking powder, salt, Italian seasoning, garlic granules, cumin, and pepper to taste. Mix well with your hands. Use a 1-ounce cookie scoop or a tablespoon to scoop out about 1 heaping tablespoon of the lentil mixture. Use your hands to squeeze and shape the mixture into tight balls about the size of walnuts. Place the balls on the prepared baking sheet.

▶ If not baking right away, cover the Lentil-Rice Balls with plastic wrap and refrigerate for several hours or overnight.

▶ Drizzle a tiny bit of olive oil on top of each ball. Bake them in the oven, turning the balls occasionally, until browned and crispy on the outside, about 30 to 35 minutes. Serve with pasta or not, but always with lots of tomato sauce.

MINI VEGAN PIZZAS

Each filling recipe makes enough for two mini-size pizzas; feel free to double or quadruple any single topping recipe or try all four!

Makes 8 mini pizzas	One recipe Easy Whole-Grain Pizza Dough (page 224) Vegan Pizza Toppings (page 161)

▶ Prepare the pizza dough, then cut the dough into eight equal pieces. Shape each piece into a smooth ball. If you are going to bake the pizzas right away, set the dough balls about 2 inches apart on a floured surface and cover lightly with plastic wrap. Let rise at room temperature for 45 minutes.

▶ If you wish to bake the pizzas later, place the balls about 2 inches apart on a well-floured baking sheet and cover well with plastic wrap. Refrigerate for several hours or overnight. When ready, take the pizza dough out of the refrigerator and let it sit at room temperature for about 15 minutes.

- Preheat the oven to 500°F. If you have a pizza stone, place it on the center rack in the oven to preheat for at least 30 minutes. If not, sprinkle a baking sheet with cornmeal and set aside.
- Working on a well-floured surface, pat out one dough ball at a time into a 6½-inch-wide circle. Top with your chosen topping, then use a pizza peel to slide your pizza directly on the hot pizza stone (or place on the baking sheet and put in the oven). Bake mini pizzas for 7 to 8 minutes, until crust is golden and the toppings are piping hot.

VEGAN PIZZA TOPPINGS

Here are four great pizzas to get you going, but I'm sure you'll soon discover that the topping ideas for vegan pizzas are simply endless!

Topping 1: Zucchini Lattice

A sophisticated-looking pizza. It looks even more impressive if you use both green and yellow zucchini and alternate colors in the lattice.

Makes enough for
2 mini pizzas

1 medium-size zucchini, preferably long
  and narrow
Kosher salt
1 large garlic clove
2 teaspoons extra virgin olive oil, plus extra
  for topping
Fresh or dried oregano

- Scrub the zucchini but do not peel. Using a mandoline or other vegetable slicer or a very sharp knife, slice the zucchini very thinly lengthwise. Place the slices in a colander in a single layer and sprinkle with salt. Set aside in the sink to drain for about 30 minutes (the zucchini will sweat out some of its moisture).

▸ Meanwhile, mash the garlic with a pinch of salt using a mortar and pestle or the flat side of a knife. Transfer to a small bowl and stir in the olive oil.

▸ Spoon out half of the garlic oil and spread evenly over the surface of the pizza crust. Pat the zucchini dry with a kitchen towel, then weave a lattice pattern on top of the garlic oil, trimming the ends as needed to fit. Sprinkle with oregano and a drizzle of olive oil. Bake according to directions on page 160.

Topping 2: Kale Kalamata

My favorite! I like to wear my "Eat More Kale" shirt while eating this one.

Makes enough for
2 mini pizzas

----

6 cups kale, hard stems removed, thinly sliced

3 tablespoons store-bought pizza sauce or
   Sneaky Momma's Tomato Sauce (page 109)

4 sun-dried tomatoes, chopped

6 Kalamata olives, pitted and sliced

Handful of pine nuts (optional)

▸ Place the kale in a steamer basket and steam until completely tender. Drain in a colander or sieve, pressing out most of the moisture.

▸ Place the kale in a bowl and toss with the pizza sauce, sun-dried tomatoes, and Kalamata olives. Spread half the kale mixture on a mini pizza crust and top with a sprinkle of pine nuts. Bake according to directions on page 160.

Topping 3: Polka-Dot Pepperoni

Guess which pizza topping my son prefers? Pepperoni, of course!

Makes enough for 2 mini pizzas	3–4 tablespoons store-bought pizza sauce or Sneaky Momma's Tomato Sauce (page 109)
	10 slices vegan pepperoni
	3 slices store-bought vegan cheese

▶ Use a 1½-inch round cookie cutter to cut four rounds out of each of the slices of cheese. Spread half the pizza sauce on each mini pizza, then top each with half the cheese and pepperoni, overlapping slightly. Bake according to directions on page 160.

Topping 4: Mixed Mushroom

The mushrooms on this pizza taste rich and meaty, their flavor intensified by sautéing until their liquid is released. Use a mixture of whichever types of fresh mushrooms you like best (I prefer a mixture of white button and cremini).

Makes enough for 2 mini pizzas	2 tablespoons extra virgin olive oil
	1 pound mixed fresh mushrooms, cleaned, stems trimmed, and sliced
	Salt
	⅛ cup chopped fresh parsley
	2 large garlic cloves, minced
	3–4 tablespoons store-bought pizza sauce or Sneaky Momma's Tomato Sauce (page 109)

▶ Heat the oil in a large nonstick sauté pan over medium-high heat. When hot, add the mushrooms and sprinkle liberally with salt. Cook, stirring frequently, until the mushrooms have given off their juices and the liquid has been cooked away, leaving the mushrooms shrunken and rich brown in color, about 10 minutes.

▸ Add the parsley and garlic and cook, stirring constantly, until the garlic has softened, about 3 minutes. Taste for salt.

▸ Top each pizza crust with half the pizza sauce and half the mushroom mixture. Bake according to directions on page 160.

PHYLLO TRIANGLES

Our family spent many years attending a Greek Orthodox church. During Lent, Orthodox Christians observe a "fast," abstaining from meat, poultry, most fish, dairy, and eggs. With the sad exception of some shellfish, this is very close to a vegan diet. As a vegan myself, I think I was probably the only person in my church who got excited over the food during Lent and felt disappointed when Easter arrived. One Easter I brought these Phyllo Triangles to a church picnic and was surprised when they were quickly devoured by everyone there— all meat eaters but for me!

The easiest way to coat the phyllo sheets with olive oil is to fill a refillable pump spray bottle with oil. Use good quality extra virgin olive oil for the best flavor.

Makes about 35 triangles

1 (½-pound) package frozen phyllo dough, thawed several hours
½ pound firm tofu
1 ½ teaspoons extra virgin olive oil
1 shallot, diced
1 garlic clove, minced
⅛ cup finely minced fresh dill
2 teaspoons freshly squeezed lemon juice

³/₄ teaspoon sea salt (or to taste)

Freshly ground black pepper

A pinch of nutmeg

Extra virgin olive oil for brushing phyllo

▸ To press the tofu, drain it, wrap it in a clean kitchen towel, and set it on a plate or cutting board. Put something heavy on top of the tofu (I use a cast-iron skillet). Press for 10 minutes. Remove the tofu from the kitchen towel and crumble it into small pieces with your fingers.

▸ Heat 1½ teaspoons olive oil in a nonstick skillet. Sauté the shallot for 1 minute, then add the garlic, crumbled tofu, and dill. Cook, stirring frequently, for another 5 minutes, until the shallot is soft and the tofu is cooked through. Remove from heat and add the lemon juice, salt, and pepper to taste. Taste for salt and lemon and add more if you wish (it should be salty and tangy). Cool to room temperature.

▸ To make the triangles, line two baking sheets with parchment paper and spray or brush with olive oil. Have ready a large pastry board or cutting board, a pizza wheel for cutting, a damp kitchen towel, plastic wrap, and a cooking oil spray pump filled with extra virgin olive oil. If you do not have a spray mister, you can use a small bowl of extra virgin olive oil and a pastry brush.

▸ Unwrap the thawed phyllo dough, then unroll just far enough to expose about 3 inches of dough. Use the pizza wheel to cut a 2½-inch-wide strip of dough, cutting through all the layers. Roll the rest of the phyllo back up in the plastic and cover with the damp cloth.

▸ Working quickly so the dough does not dry out, lay out a single strip of phyllo. Spray or brush lightly with oil, then top with another layer of phyllo, spray again, and add one more layer of phyllo. Spray with oil.

▸ Place 2 teaspoons of filling on the bottom corner of the phyllo strip. Fold the filling up in the dough as if folding up a flag, touching the bottom corner to the opposite side, then folding up, then folding the other corner to the opposite side, and repeating all the way to the top to form a small triangle bundle. Place the triangles on the prepared baking sheet, seam side down, and brush or spray with olive oil. Keep the prepared triangles covered with plastic wrap so they do not dry out.

▸ Repeat with all the remaining phyllo dough and filling (I like to create an assembly line of four to six phyllo strips at a time). When finished, double wrap the two baking sheets with plastic wrap and place in the refrigerator overnight or until needed.

▸ When ready to bake, preheat the oven to 375°F. Take the baking sheet from the refrigerator and remove the plastic wrap. Bake for 20 minutes, or until golden and crisp. Cool on a wire rack.

VARIATION: Spinach Triangles: Ah, my favorite: steam 1 (5-ounce) package of baby spinach (about 3 cups) until tender. Drain thoroughly in a fine mesh sieve or colander, pressing excess moisture out of the spinach with the back of a spoon. Place the cooked spinach on a chopping block and chop fine. Fold the spinach into the prepared tofu mixture and proceed with the recipe.

VARIATION: Phyllo Bundles: One tester reported that her daughter thought the triangles had "too much crust" (those darned crusts will get you every time). So for Shannon, here's an easy little bundle with less than half the phyllo: cut the phyllo into 4½-inch squares. Brush one square with olive oil, then lay another square on top, tilted slightly. Fill the center with the tofu mixture and bring the edges up, pinching them together with the edges of phyllo poking up like a pouch. Bake for about 20 minutes, until golden and crisp.

PUPS IN BLANKETS

You can assemble these in the morning or the night before. If your children like to help in the kitchen, let them flatten out the dough with a rolling pin and help roll up their own little veggie pups. They are perfect with ketchup or mustard on the side for dipping.

Makes 5

$^1/_3$ cup plain, unsweetened soymilk

$^3/_4$ teaspoon apple cider vinegar

1 cup all-purpose flour

1 teaspoon baking powder

$^1/_4$ teaspoon baking soda

$^1/_4$ teaspoon kosher salt

3 tablespoons wheat germ

$^1/_4$ cup nonhydrogenated margarine, chilled

5 soy hot dogs

▸ If you are baking these right away, preheat the oven to 375°F.

▸ Line a baking sheet with parchment paper, spray with nonstick spray, and set aside.

▸ Mix the soymilk and apple cider vinegar and set aside.

▸ Whisk the flour, baking powder, baking soda, salt, and wheat germ together in a medium mixing bowl. Cut in the margarine with your fingers or a pastry cutter, until the mixture resembles coarse meal. Add the soymilk mixture and stir until a dough forms.

▸ Turn dough out onto a lightly floured surface and knead four or five times, just enough to incorporate any loose pieces of dough. Add more flour as needed to keep the dough from sticking. Roll the dough out into a 10-inch square using a lightly floured rolling pin and cut into five 2-inch strips.

▸ Working with one strip at a time, place a soy hot dog at a slight angle at the base of a strip of dough. Roll the dog up in the dough so that the dough overlaps along the length of the hot dog and covers the dog from end to end, leaving just the tips of the hot dog exposed. Press the seam and edges gently to secure. Place the pups seam side down on the baking sheet. Repeat with remaining dogs and dough.

▸ At this point, the pups can be covered in plastic wrap and refrigerated until the morning. When ready to bake, remove the pups from the refrigerator and preheat the oven to 375°F.

▸ Bake until the pups are warmed through and the dough is browned on the bottom, 15 to 18 minutes.

VARIATION: Piroshki are small Russian hand pies, usually filled with potato and onion, cooked kasha (buckwheat), or ground meat. We like to use leftover mashed potatoes seasoned with plenty of black pepper to make a simple piroshki filling:

▸ Roll out the dough and cut into six rectangles. Place a small, long mound of cooled mashed potatoes or other filling in the center and seal completely in dough. Follow baking instructions above.

QUINOA AMARANTH TIMBALES

You will need several small cups or molds to shape these timbales into individual servings. For the Quinoa Amaranth Timbale pictured in the insert, I used the small dressing container in my Laptop Lunch Box to make three mini timbales and lined them up side by side in the larger lunch container; you can also use the medium-size container to make one larger timbale, or use ramekins or teacups to make round or dome shapes.

Be sure to rinse the quinoa well under running water using a fine sieve; quinoa has a bitter surface coating (a kind of natural insect repellent) that must be rinsed off before use.

And the answer is yes—the timbale does hold its shape, even in the swinging lunch box of a seven-year-old!

Makes 5

Zest and juice of 1 orange
1 teaspoon canola oil
1/2 a small onion, finely diced
1/2 teaspoon cumin
1/4 teaspoon salt
1/4 cup amaranth
1/2 cup quinoa, well rinsed and drained
1/4 teaspoon cinnamon
1 tablespoon pine nuts (optional)
5 dried apricot halves, finely diced

▶ Zest the orange and set zest aside. Juice the orange into a 2-cup liquid measuring cup, then fill the cup with water to equal 1½ cups. Set aside.

▶ Heat the oil in a small saucepan. Sauté the onion until tender, about 5 minutes. Add the cumin and cook for 30 seconds, until the cumin is fragrant. Add the orange juice mixture and salt and bring to a boil. Remove from heat and slowly add the amaranth, whisking constantly. Add the quinoa and cinnamon and whisk to combine.

▸ Return the pan to the heat. When the water boils, turn the heat to low, cover, and let cook on low heat until all the liquid has been absorbed and the grains are tender, about 25 minutes.

▸ Meanwhile, toast the pine nuts in a dry skillet over medium heat, stirring constantly until lightly toasted, about 4 minutes (watch the pine nuts carefully, as they burn easily).

▸ When the grains are done, stir in the dried apricot, pine nuts, and orange zest. Stir briskly until well incorporated.

▸ Spray your mold(s) with nonstick spray. Pack the quinoa mixture firmly into the mold, then immediately turn it out onto a serving dish or container, tapping on the bottom to help it release.

RED RICE AND BLACK BEANS

Cooking the rice in tomato or vegetable juice adds vibrant flavor and color.

Makes 4 servings

1/2 tablespoon extra virgin olive oil

1/2 a small onion, diced

1/4 red bell pepper, diced

1 celery stalk, diced

1 garlic clove, minced

1/2 teaspoon ground cumin

1/2 teaspoon paprika

1 cup uncooked long-grain rice (brown or white, your choice)

1/4 teaspoon dried oregano

3/4 cup R. W. Knudsen Low Sodium Very Veggie Juice or other low-sodium tomato juice

Kosher salt

1 (15-ounce) can black beans, drained
and rinsed

▸ Heat the olive oil in a large saucepan set over medium high heat. Add the onion, red bell pepper, and celery and sauté, stirring frequently, until the onion softens and just begins to brown, about 5 minutes. Add the garlic, cumin, and paprika and cook, stirring constantly, for another 30 seconds. Add the rice and oregano and cook, stirring, for another minute.

▸ Add the vegetable juice and 1¼ cups water. Turn the heat to high, bring to a boil, then lower the heat and simmer, covered, until the rice is tender and the water is absorbed, about 25 to 30 minutes for white rice, an hour for brown. Add salt to taste.

▸ Stir the beans directly into the rice, or keep the beans and rice separated with a thin spatula as you fill the serving dish to create a colorful effect.

SAVORY AUTUMN LEAF PIES

These little pies are admittedly a bit of work to produce, but worth it if the equinox is a special holiday in your household. For a simpler meal, you can bake it as one big pie (see first variation below). The pastries can be assembled the night before and baked in the morning.

Makes about
24 leaf pies

Special equipment you will need:
2 (4-inch) oak- and maple leaf–shaped
cookie cutters

For the vegetable filling:
2 large carrots, peeled and diced in $\frac{1}{4}$-inch
pieces (about 1 cup)
1 small parsnip or golden beet, peeled and
diced in $\frac{1}{4}$-inch pieces (about $\frac{1}{2}$ cup)
2 medium-size new potatoes, peeled and
diced into $\frac{1}{2}$-inch pieces (about 2 cups)
2 garlic cloves, left whole and unpeeled
4 sprigs fresh thyme
2 tablespoons extra virgin olive oil
$\frac{1}{2}$ teaspoon kosher salt

For the barley poppy seed crust:
2 cups all-purpose flour
1 cup barley flour
$\frac{1}{2}$ teaspoon baking soda
$\frac{1}{2}$ teaspoon kosher salt
1 teaspoon poppy seeds
$\frac{1}{2}$ cup canola oil, chilled in the freezer for at
least 30 minutes
$\frac{1}{2}$ cup ice water
1 tablespoon apple cider vinegar

- Preheat the oven to 425°F. Line a baking sheet with parchment paper.
- Place the diced vegetables on the baking sheet with the garlic cloves and thyme. Drizzle with the olive oil and salt, and toss to coat. Spread the vegetables out in one even layer.
- Roast for 25 to 30 minutes or until tender, stirring occasionally to ensure even roasting. Remove from oven and allow to cool slightly. Remove the thyme sprigs.
- When the vegetables are cool enough to touch, squeeze the roasted garlic out of its skin. Mash the garlic well with the back of a fork, then toss thoroughly with the vegetables until well distributed. Set vegetables aside while you prepare the crust.
- Line two baking sheets with parchment paper and spray with nonstick spray. Place a small bowl of water and a brush next to the baking sheet. Set aside.
- In a medium mixing bowl, combine the flour, barley flour, baking soda, salt, and poppy seeds and whisk to combine. Drizzle in the canola oil and toss with your fingers until the oil is incorporated and the flour has formed small to medium-size clumps. Mix the ice water with the cider vinegar and drizzle it into the flour, stirring with your fingers until the dough holds together.
- Turn the dough out onto a lightly floured surface. Knead a few times, then divide the dough into three pieces, covering two with plastic as you roll out the first one.
- Lightly flour your work surface and roll the dough as thinly as possible—at least 1/8 inch. Use the cookie cutters to cut out leaf shapes.
- To make the pies, place one leaf on the baking sheet and top with 1 tablespoon of vegetable filling. Pick up a matching leaf shape, brush the edges with water and place on top of the filled leaf. Press the edges together with your fingers, then pick the pie up and pinch the edges shut all the way around the pie. Repeat with the remaining dough and filling.

▸ Brush or spray the pies lightly with olive oil. If not baking right away, cover the baking sheets with plastic wrap and refrigerate several hours or overnight.

▸ When ready to bake, preheat the oven to 375°F. Poke two small holes in the top of each pie with a cake tester or toothpick. Bake for 20 minutes, until golden brown (up to 30 minutes if coming from the refrigerator).

VARIATION: For an easier meal, line a 9-inch pie pan with the barley crust or your favorite piecrust, fill with the vegetable mixture, and top with piecrust. Cut a small slit in the center of the pie to release steam. Bake at 375°F for 35 to 40 minutes. Cut in wedges to serve.

VARIATION: If you're lucky enough to have a child who likes kale (and that is lucky—kale is an exceptionally nutritious green rich in calcium and many other vitamins and minerals), steam one bunch of chopped kale until tender, toss with 1 tablespoon soy sauce, and add it to the vegetable mixture. Bake as individual hand pies or one big pie.

VARIATION: "Leaves Falling in the Mud": Although they taste very good plain, I like to dip these little hand pies in store-bought tamarind chutney.

SPANISH EMPANADAS

If you're feeling particularly adventurous, try adding some sautéed onions, chopped green olives, and raisins to the veggie meat (a traditional combination in Argentina).

Makes 4–5 empanadas	1 (16-ounce) package of vegan taco-flavored ground beef
	1 recipe Easy Piecrust (page 211)

▸ Line a baking sheet with parchment paper and spray with nonstick spray. Have a small bowl of water ready

▸ To form the empanadas, divide the piecrust into four equal pieces. Lightly flour a work surface and roll the dough out with a rolling pin to about ⅛ inch thick. Cut the pastry into a 7-inch-wide circle (use a small plate or saucer to help guide you). Cover half of the pastry with 4 to 5 tablespoon of veggie meat, leaving about ½ inch uncovered around the edges.

▸ Dip your fingers in water and moisten the edges of the pastry, then fold over the dough. Use a fork to crimp the edges all the way around and use a sharp knife to cut decorative slits in the top of the dough. Repeat with the remaining pastry and filling. You may wish to gather the pastry scraps together to make one final empanada. Spray or brush them with olive oil. At this point, the empanadas may be refrigerated for several hours or overnight.

▸ When ready to bake, preheat the oven to 400°F. Bake for 25 minutes, until lightly browned and warmed through.

SUNNY WHOLE-GRAIN SUSHI

As I was experimenting with healthier sushi rolls, I found that brown rice alone did not get sticky enough to spread well on nori like traditional white sushi rice. I solved the problem by adding tasty millet and tiny amaranth to my brown rice. I found that cooking the three grains together resulted in perfect sushi rice, along with extra flavor and nutrition. A hint of lemon and the crunch of sunflower seeds add flavor and interest.

When it comes time to fill and roll your sushi, there are dozens of delightful vegan fillings you can choose from. Avocado is our favorite, but you also might like blanched asparagus, red bell pepper strips, cucumber, grilled shiitake, or even fresh mango (see page 181 for more sushi filling ideas). Pack with a small container of regular soy sauce or refreshing, lower-sodium Ponzu Sauce (page 177) for dipping.

Makes 4 rolls,
to serve 2

$3/4$ cup short-grain brown rice

$1/8$ cup millet

$1/8$ cup amaranth

1 teaspoon fresh lemon zest

$1/8$ cup sunflower seeds

4 sushi nori sheets (sheets of dried, toasted nori seaweed)

Avocado slices or other filling of your choice

▸ Put the rice, millet, and amaranth into a medium pot and add $1\frac{1}{2}$ cups water. Bring to a boil, reduce the heat to low, and cook, covered, for 35 minutes. Remove pan from heat and let sit, still covered, for another 10 minutes.

▸ Transfer the rice mixture to a large mixing bowl. Stir in the lemon zest and sunflower seeds with a wooden rice paddle or spoon, tossing the rice with light strokes to aerate and cool it. Set the rice mixture aside to cool completely.

▸ When the rice is cool, spread one-quarter of the mixture on a sheet of nori laid out on a sushi rolling mat (keep a small bowl of fresh water handy to dip your fingers in to keep the rice from sticking). Leave a 1-inch strip at the top of the nori sheet uncovered. Arrange the avocado or other filling down the center of the rice. Use your fingers to lightly moisten the top strip of nori with a dab of water, then use the rolling mat to roll your sushi up and seal it shut.

▸ Transfer the roll to a cutting board and cut into six pieces with a sharp knife, wiping the knife with a damp cloth between cuts.

PONZU SAUCE

This makes a refreshing, lower-sodium alternative to plain soy sauce for dipping sushi.

Makes about ¼ cup	1 tablespoon low-sodium soy sauce
	1 tablespoon brown rice vinegar
	1 tablespoon mirin (sweet Japanese cooking wine)
	1 tablespoon freshly squeezed lime juice

▸ Combine all ingredients. Adjust seasonings to suit your taste.

SUSHI ROLLS

Making your own sushi can seem daunting at first. But once you get the hang of it, the process becomes simple and straightforward: rice is cooked, then tossed with a mixture of sugar, salt, and vinegar until cool. The rice is spread on a sheet of nori seaweed; the desired filling is set in place, and the roll is wrapped up and sliced.

I recommend making smaller, narrow-rolled sushi (hosomaki-zushi) for a child-size mouth; sushi rolls should be eaten in one bite. The nori seaweed is very hard to bite through, and a half-bitten sushi will fall apart.

Look for supplies and ingredients at Asian markets and some grocery and natural food stores.

Makes 3–4 servings	*Special equipment you will need:*

Special equipment you will need:

Wide, shallow wooden bowl (or a *hangiri*) for mixing the rice

Wooden rice paddle or wooden spoon

Fan (electric or handheld)

Bamboo rolling mat

2 cups uncooked sushi rice (short-grain sticky rice)

3 tablespoons brown rice vinegar

3 tablespoons mirin (sweet Japanese cooking wine)

3 tablespoons sugar

1 tablespoon coarse sea salt or kosher salt

Sushi nori sheets (sheets of dried, toasted nori seaweed)

Vegan Sushi Fillings (page 181)

Soy sauce for dipping

Wasabi (hot Japanese horseradish paste, optional)
Pickled ginger (optional)

- Rinse the rice several times in cold water until water runs clear. Put rice in a medium pot and cover with water. Let soak for 30 minutes.
- Drain the water, then add fresh water in a ratio of 1 cup uncooked rice to $\frac{1}{5}$ cup water. Bring water to a boil, reduce heat, and simmer, covered, for 20 minutes (or use a rice cooker if you have one).
- Remove from heat and let sit, still covered, for 10 minutes. The resulting rice should be sticky, slightly wet, and shiny.
- While the rice is cooking, make the vinegar dressing by stirring together the vinegar, mirin, sugar, and salt until the sugar dissolves. Avoid using metal utensils when making sushi vinegar and sushi rice; the vinegar may react with the metal and create a disturbing taste. Set aside the sushi vinegar and prepare your fillings (see list of ideas on page 181).
- Fill another small bowl with 1 cup water and 2 tablespoons vinegar. This vinegared water is used to wet the mixing tub. Moisten your fingers to prevent the rice from sticking while you roll the sushi.
- Wet a wide, shallow wooden bowl or Japanese hangiri (wooden mixing tub) with water and pour off excess. Wet the tub a second time with some of the vinegared water and wipe off any excess (this will keep the rice from sticking to the tub).
- When the rice is done, heap the cooked rice in the center of the damp tub. Pour the vinegar dressing over the peak of the mound of rice. With a rice paddle or wooden spoon, cut through the mound of rice; toss with horizontal, cutting strokes.
- Use a fan to cool the rice as you toss. If you're coordinated, you can toss with one hand and fan with the other, but I find an electric desktop fan works well. Cooling and tossing in this way gives

the rice good flavor, texture, and gloss. Once the rice has cooled to room temperature, it is ready to use. If you are not using the rice immediately, cover with a damp cloth. Do not refrigerate sushi rice; if it becomes too cold it hardens.

- Now, you're ready to roll sushi! For futomaki-zushi (thick-rolled sushi), use a whole sheet of nori. For smaller hosomaki-zushi (narrow-rolled sushi), cut a sheet of nori in half with kitchen shears.

- Place the nori sheet at the base of the bamboo rolling mat. Wet your hands with vinegared water and scoop up a ball of sushi rice. Spread the rice evenly over the nori, leaving a ¾- to 1-inch strip at the top of the nori sheet uncovered. Remember, too little rice is better than too much; too much rice could break holes in the nori or cause the roll to split open.

- Arrange the filling ingredients in the center of the sushi rice. Use your fingers to lightly moisten the top strip of nori with vinegared water; this will seal the nori roll. Immediately pick up the end of the rolling mat and roll everything together forward, tightly wrapping rice and nori around the fillings. Press on the mat to shape and seal the roll.

- Unroll the mat and place the sushi roll on a cutting board with the seam facing down. Cut roll into six pieces with a very sharp knife, wiping the knife with a damp cloth in between cuts.

- Serve your sushi with soy sauce, wasabi, and pickled ginger. Sushi should ideally be eaten the same day it is made.

Vegan Sushi Fillings

Here are some vegan sushi filling ideas to get you started. Mix-and-match, use your imagination, and go sushi crazy!

- avocado
- peeled, seeded cucumber
- strips of fried tofu
- umeboshi (salty, pickled Japanese plums)
- grilled fresh shiitake mushrooms
- blanched carrot strips
- blanched asparagus spears
- mango slices and avocado
- fried tempeh strips
- blanched spinach, drained and chopped with toasted sesame oil and toasted pine nuts
- red bell pepper strips, raw or roasted
- blanched zucchini strips
- blanched green beans
- radish sprouts
- raw spinach with tofu and grated carrot
- *takuan* (pickled daikon radish)
- *kampyo* (strips of gourd simmered in sweetened soy sauce, available in cans or refrigerated packets)
- strips of grilled eggplant

TOFU FISH STICKS

Kelp granules give these tofu sticks a hint of fishy flavor. They can be found in shaker containers at health food stores or online at www.veganessentials.com. Sprinkle them on any food for a low-sodium salt alternative; they are a good source of iodine.

Makes 4 servings

⅔ cup fine cornmeal (or all-purpose flour)

⅔ cup sliced almonds

2 teaspoons paprika

2 teaspoons kelp granules

2 teaspoons salt

½ teaspoon onion powder

½ teaspoon garlic powder

¼ teaspoon dried dill weed

Freshly ground black pepper

⅔ cup plain, unsweetened soymilk

1 pound firm tofu, drained

Extra virgin olive oil

1 lemon, cut in wedges for squeezing

▸ Preheat the oven to 400°F. Line a baking sheet with parchment paper and coat it with olive oil. Set aside.

▸ Combine the cornmeal or flour, sliced almonds, paprika, kelp, salt, onion powder, garlic powder, dill weed, and pepper to taste in a blender. Blend on high until most of the almonds have been turned into a coarse meal, with a few larger pieces of almond remaining. Pour the mixture into a wide baking dish or pie plate.

▸ Place the plain soymilk into a bowl and set next to the cornmeal mixture.

▸ With a sharp knife, cut the tofu into even slices just under ½ inch wide. Cut the slices into fish stick dimensions or use a fish-shaped cookie cutter to cut out tofu fish. Working with one piece at a time, dip the tofu into the soymilk, then toss gently in the cornmeal mixture to coat evenly. Place on the prepared baking sheet. When all the tofu fish are on the baking sheet, sprinkle them with olive oil.

▸ Bake for 15 minutes, then turn the tofu over and bake for an additional 15 minutes, or until crispy (if making Tater Tots to go with the fish sticks, place them on the baking sheet for the last 15 minutes). Squeeze some lemon juice evenly over the tofu fish and serve.

HOW MUCH TO PACK

Here are comments I received from two readers of my online site, Vegan LunchBox.com, in the same week: "Are you sure your child isn't eating too much? Your meals look big for a child in first grade!" and "Does your son really eat so little? My little one could eat TWO of those lunches and still be ravenous!"

It's hard to know how much to pack at times. Packing too much can make a lunch look overwhelming to a small child and can lead to a lot of wasted food. But, of course, we don't want to pack so little that our son or daughter doesn't get full.

Only you know your children well enough to determine how much will be enough for them. One trick I use is to imagine my son's dinner plate when I'm stocking his lunch box. Since I eat with him every day at the table, I have a fairly good idea of how much he will eat from a plate of food. I try to aim for that amount when packing his lunch containers.

Most of the kids I know have appetites that fluctuate over time. Some days they can't seem to get enough; other days they just pick at their food. If you consistently keep your kitchen (and lunch box) stocked with healthy foods and keep out unhealthy choices, this fluctuation shouldn't be a cause for worry. Most kids, given a wide variety of whole, healthy foods, will naturally adjust how much they eat to meet their needs.

Oh, and don't forget to have a healthy after-school snack ready when your children get home. No matter how good lunch was, by the afternoon they'll be ready to refuel!

WHEAT GLUTEN POT ROAST AND GRAVY

Wheat gluten, also knows as seitan, is made from the protein of wheat after the starch has been rinsed away. It has a chewy, "meaty" texture, and because this pot roast is entirely soy-free, it makes a great alternative to store-bought meat analogues for those with soy allergies or intolerances.

Wheat Gluten Pot Roast is simple to prepare using vital wheat gluten powder, available at most health food stores.

Makes 4 servings with leftovers for lunch the next day

2 vegetarian beef-flavored bullion cubes (Celifibr brand is all-natural and soy-free. If you can't find it locally, you can order it online at www.glutenfreemall.com)

1 teaspoon kosher salt

1 1/4 cups vital wheat gluten powder

1/4 cup ground walnuts (use a food processor to grind to a coarse meal)

2 tablespoons nutritional yeast flakes

1/2 teaspoon onion powder

1/2 teaspoon garlic powder

3 tablespoons extra virgin olive oil

1 teaspoon plus 2 tablespoons tomato paste

1 teaspoon Marmite or other yeast extract

1 large onion, sliced

1 celery stalk, chopped

2 large garlic cloves, minced

1/2 cup dry red wine

1 cup sliced button or cremini mushrooms

1/8 cup uncooked red lentils

4 sprigs of fresh thyme

4 large carrots, peeled and cut into
2-inch chunks
Salt and freshly ground black pepper

- Bring 4 cups of water to a boil. Remove from heat and stir in the two bullion cubes and salt. Let the cubes dissolve completely as you prepare the pot roast.
- In a medium mixing bowl, stir together the vital wheat gluten powder, ground walnuts, nutritional yeast, onion powder, and garlic powder. Measure out 1 cup of the bullion broth and set the rest aside. To the 1 cup of broth, add 1 tablespoon olive oil, 1 teaspoon tomato paste, and the yeast extract. Add the liquid to the vital wheat gluten and stir together until the mixture forms a dough. Knead in the bowl just enough to form into a smooth loaf. Sprinkle the loaf evenly with salt and pepper to taste.
- In a large Dutch oven or saucepan, heat the remaining 2 tablespoons of olive oil. When hot, add the pot roast loaf and sear on all sides until dark brown. Remove from the heat and set aside on a plate.
- Add the onions and celery to the saucepan and cook, stirring frequently, until the onions are soft and beginning to brown, about 5 minutes. Add the minced garlic and cook, stirring, for 1 more minute, until the garlic is softened but not brown.
- Add the red wine and the remaining 2 tablespoons tomato paste. Stir until the tomato paste is dissolved, then cook at a lively simmer until the wine has completely evaporated, about 3 minutes. Add the remaining bullion broth, mushrooms, red lentils, and thyme sprigs. Place the pot roast in the center of the broth and arrange the carrots around the sides.
- Turn the heat to the lowest possible setting. You want the broth hot enough to be sending up a bubble every so often, but never

boiling. Simmer like this for 45 minutes, then turn the pot roast over and simmer for another 45 minutes.

▸ Remove the pot roast and all but one of the carrot chunks from the broth. Cover the roast and carrots with foil or an inverted bowl to stay warm as you prepare the gravy.

▸ Remove the thyme sprigs from the broth, then transfer the broth and vegetables to a blender and blend until completely smooth. Return the gravy to a small saucepan and warm over low heat. Taste for salt and pepper and serve hot.

▸ This meaty, soy-free pot roast makes a great dinner, served with cooked carrots, peas, and mashed potatoes. Leftovers can be served for lunch in at least three different ways:

VARIATIONS: How to Pack a Pot Roast

- Cut slices of pot roast into bite-size pieces and serve as finger food with a small container of ketchup for dipping.
- Cut into thicker slices and use as a sandwich filling with Vegenaise, ketchup, and fresh veggies.
- Dice some pot roast and mix it in with leftover gravy. Pack the hot gravy in a preheated insulated food jar alongside some split Spelt Biscuits (page 216). At lunch, pour the gravy over the biscuits for some hot, "beefy" biscuits and gravy.

WILD RICE PILAF

This lemony wild rice dish, flecked with sweet green peas, corn, and bits of toasted pecan, is wonderful served at room temperature, making it perfect to take with you to a Thanksgiving dinner or veggie potluck.

Wild rice is now being sold fully cooked in vacuum-sealed packages (I get mine from Trader Joe's). These packages are a quick and convenient way to eat this usually long-cooking grain. If you can't find precooked wild rice in your area, you can still buy dried wild rice and cook it according to the directions below.

Makes 6–8 servings

½ cup chopped pecans

2 cups cooked wild rice, or 1 cup dried

1 tablespoon extra virgin olive oil

1 shallot, finely minced

1 cup uncooked long-grain white rice

1 teaspoon salt

1 cup mixed frozen peas and corn

Juice and zest of one lemon

Freshly ground pepper

▸ Preheat the oven to 350°F. Place the chopped pecans on a baking sheet and toast, shaking the pan one or two times, for 10 minutes, until the pecans are toasted and fragrant. Set aside.

▸ If using precooked rice, skip ahead to the next step. To cook wild rice, bring a large pot of lightly salted water to a boil. Add the wild rice and reduce heat. Simmer until the wild rice is tender but not split, about 45 to 50 minutes. Drain the rice and set aside.

▸ In a medium saucepan set over medium-high heat, warm the olive oil. When hot, add the shallot and cook, stirring, until the shallot is soft, about 2 minutes. Add the white rice and salt and cook, stirring, until rice just starts to turn translucent, about 3 minutes. Pour in 1½ cups water. Bring to a boil, turn the heat to low, and cover. Steam until the rice is tender, about 20 minutes.

▸ When the rice is done, turn off the heat. Open the lid and sprinkle the frozen mixed vegetables on top of the cooked rice. Cover again and allow the vegetables to steam until just tender, about 5 minutes. Transfer the rice and vegetables to a serving dish and stir in the wild rice, lemon juice and zest, and pepper to taste. Top with the toasted pecans.

VEGGIE AND BEAN SIDES

ADZUKI BEANS WITH PICKLED GINGER

Adzuki beans are small, reddish beans with a hint of sweetness. They can be found in many Asian markets and health food stores. In Japanese cuisine, they are often made into a sweet paste and used to make cakes and sweets.

I love to serve this dish alongside sushi as well as Musubi (page 79). The beans add protein to the meal and highlight the flavor of the pickled ginger that we like to nibble on between sushi bites.

Makes 3 servings

1 (15-ounce) can adzuki beans, rinsed and drained

3 tablespoons diced pickled ginger, with juice (preferably all-natural)

2 teaspoons soy sauce

1/2 teaspoon mirin (sweet Japanese cooking wine)

1 scallion, white and part of the green, minced

Toasted sesame seeds for garnish

- Combine the adzuki beans, pickled ginger, soy sauce, mirin, and scallion and toss together gently with a spatula. Refrigerate until cold. Taste for salt and serve cold or at room temperature, sprinkled with toasted sesame seeds.

ALMOND BUTTERED SWEET POTATOES

I'm still swooning over these rich, creamy sweet potatoes. I like to sprinkle a bit of ground flaxseed over mine and enjoy them for breakfast, but they're perfectly delectable just as they are any time of day.

Makes 2 servings

1 medium-size sweet potato or garnet yam, baked until soft (see page 151)
1 tablespoon freshly squeezed orange juice
2 tablespoons light brown sugar (optional)
½ teaspoon cinnamon
A pinch of nutmeg
1 tablespoon creamy almond butter

- Peel and chop the baked sweet potato. Place sweet potato chunks in a food processor along with the orange juice, brown sugar, cinnamon, and nutmeg and process until creamy and smooth.
- Scrape the sweet potato mixture into a small saucepan and heat gently on the stove over medium heat until warmed through, stirring frequently. Remove from heat and stir in the almond butter until well combined. Taste for seasonings and add a bit more juice or sweetener, if desired. Serve warm or at room temperature.

BEST BRUSSELS SPROUTS

The name says it all! These sweet-and-sour sprouts are wonderful hot or at room temperature. We usually can't stop ourselves from eating them straight from the pan before they make it to the table.

Makes 4 servings

1 pound fresh brussels sprouts, cleaned, trimmed, and cut in half

2 tablespoons olive oil (or 1 tablespoon olive oil and 1 tablespoon margarine)

Salt

$3/4$ cup vegetable stock (or water)

2 tablespoons sugar

2 tablespoons apple cider vinegar

Freshly ground black pepper

▸ Heat the oil or oil and margarine in a sauté pan or well-seasoned cast-iron skillet over medium-high heat. When hot, add the brussels sprouts and sprinkle with salt to taste. Sauté, stirring occasionally, until the sprouts begin to turn golden, about 5 to 10 minutes.

▸ Add $1/2$ cup of the stock or water and bring to a boil. Lower the heat and simmer, covered with the lid left slightly ajar, until the brussels sprouts are almost completely tender and the stock or water has been cooked away, about 10 minutes.

▸ Remove the lid and add the last $1/4$ cup of stock or water, the sugar, and the apple cider vinegar. Cook at a lively simmer, stirring occasionally, until the liquid is reduced to a syrup, about 5 minutes. Taste for salt and season with pepper as desired. Serve hot or at room temperature.

BROCCOLI PICCATA

Your broccoli is crying out for lemon and capers, did you know? This simple sauce packs a big flavor that is perfect with steamed broccoli.

Makes 4 servings

1 large bunch of broccoli, rinsed and cut
    into florets
2 tablespoons olive oil
½ teaspoon minced garlic
2 tablespoons freshly squeezed lemon juice
2 tablespoons capers, rinsed and drained
1 teaspoon cornstarch mixed with
    2 tablespoons water (or vegetable broth)
Salt and freshly ground black pepper
1 tablespoon minced fresh parsley (optional)

▸ Put the broccoli in a steamer basket and steam until tender.

▸ Meanwhile, heat the olive oil in a small saucepan over medium-high heat. When the oil is hot, add the garlic and cook, stirring constantly, for about 30 seconds, just long enough for the garlic to soften without turning brown. Add the lemon juice, capers, and cornstarch mixture and cook, stirring, until thickened, about 2 minutes.

▸ Remove the sauce from the heat and add salt and freshly ground black pepper to taste (taste it before adding salt—capers are salty).

▸ Place the steamed broccoli in a serving dish and pour the sauce evenly over the top. Garnish with a sprinkle of parsley if desired.

▸ Serve immediately or place a serving of the broccoli and sauce in a covered container for the lunch box. This dish is good served warm or at room temperature.

CALABACITA CON ELOTE

In parts of Mexico, cooks make their own mild vinegars using sweet fruit like pineapple. This flavorful salad of zucchini and corn has a simple dressing of fruity Late Harvest Riesling Vinegar, available at gourmet markets and online.

Look for Mexican zucchini (calabacita) at grocery stores and farmers' markets. Regular zucchini makes a fine substitute.

Makes 6 to 8 servings

1 tablespoon canola oil

1/4 of a red onion, finely diced

2 Mexican or regular zucchini, cut into a 1/2-inch dice

1 cup frozen corn, thawed

1 tablespoon Late Harvest Riesling Vinegar

1/2 teaspoon dried marjoram

1/4 teaspoon kosher salt (or to taste)

Freshly ground black pepper

▶ In a large nonstick or cast-iron skillet, heat the oil over medium heat. When hot, add the onion and cook, stirring, until the onion is just starting to soften, about 2 minutes. Add the zucchini and cook, stirring, until the zucchini is warm and just barely starting to soften, about 3 minutes.

▶ Remove from heat and stir in the corn. In a small cup, stir together the vinegar, marjoram, and salt and pour over the zucchini mixture. Toss well, add salt to taste, and sprinkle with a generous amount of black pepper. Set aside to cool. Serve cold or at room temperature.

CHEESY ROASTED CHICKPEAS

These chickpeas (also called garbanzo beans) fill the house with an amazing, tantalizing smell like hot buttered popcorn as they roast. In fact, I like to make them on family movie nights and serve them in place of regular popcorn. They are chewy on the outside and soft on the inside, and nutritional yeast flakes give them a cheesy flavor.

Makes about 1½ cups

1 (15-ounce) can chickpeas, rinsed and drained

1 tablespoon canola oil

1½ teaspoons nutritional yeast flakes

½ teaspoon kosher salt (or to taste)

▸ Preheat the oven to 400°F. Line a baking sheet with parchment paper.

▸ Toss the chickpeas in a medium bowl with the oil, yeast flakes, and salt. Spread in a single layer on the baking sheet.

▸ Roast for 30 minutes, stirring occasionally, until golden and slightly crispy. Once cooled, store in an airtight container.

VARIATION: *Fast Cheesy Chickpeas:* When you just can't wait: open a can of chickpeas, rinse and drain, pat dry, then sprinkle with the nutritional yeast and salt. *Voilà!*

LET'S HEAR IT FOR LEGUMES!

Whenever I spend time sitting at a vegan information table or talking to others about veganism, I often hear words such as these: "I couldn't be vegan, my body needs protein." . . . "I couldn't be vegan, it's too expensive." . . . "I couldn't be vegan, that 'rabbit food' would never fill me up."

What wonderful food family is the perfect answer to all these problems and more?

LEGUMES! That's right, legumes, also known as beans, peas, pulses, and lentils.

Legumes are an excellent source of low-fat plant protein. They are absolutely loaded with healthy fiber, antioxidants, folate, iron, and magnesium. They are hearty, filling, immensely satisfying, and supercheap to boot!

"But my son/daughter/husband/great aunt doesn't like beans." Are you sure? There are hundreds of different varieties of legumes out there and an endless number of ways to enjoy them. It's worth experimenting to find some that you enjoy. We eat beans almost every day and never seem to run out of new ways to prepare them. We mash them into spreads and dips, roll them up in wraps, bake them, stew them, shake them into salads, cook them in soups, and fry them into burger patties.

If the long soaking and cooking time is putting you off, remember that canned beans, although more expensive than dried, are quick and convenient. Black-eyed peas and baby lima beans are available precooked and frozen. Dried split peas cook quickly, as do lentils (lentils are also a great source of iron). Indian dahls are split, husked legumes that cook in a flash and are easy to digest.

Oh, but beans make you (ahem) gassy? Well, if you share the same sense of humor as my seven-year old, that's just a bonus. If not, remember that the gassiness does diminish over time if you continue to eat beans on a regular basis. Start with small portions and build up. Try taking a walk after dinner to aid digestion. There are also digestive enzyme tablets on the market that can help.

Legumes truly deserve to have a place of honor at every vegan table! Serve them up each day and you'll be providing your family with a filling, satisfying source of protein, fiber, and nutrition.

CHRISTMAS LIMAS WITH CHESTNUTS AND BRUSSELS SPROUTS

This is a festive celebration dish for the holidays, filled with sweet chestnuts and hearty Christmas lima beans. Christmas limas are also called chestnut limas, because they have the nutty flavor and potato-ey texture of a chestnut. They are lovely, large beans with white and burgundy swirls that you can still see after the beans are cooked.

The brussels sprouts are finely shredded and almost disappear into the dish—a nice way to get sneaky with those sprouts if your family doesn't take to them whole.

Makes 6 servings

1 cup dried Christmas lima beans

2 tablespoons olive oil

8 fresh brussels sprouts, cleaned, ends removed, and leaves removed and finely shredded

1 (7-ounce) package vacuum-packed whole chestnuts (or 20 fresh chestnuts, roasted and peeled)

3 tablespoons golden brown sugar

1 tablespoon apple cider vinegar

Salt and freshly ground black pepper

▶ Soak the lima beans overnight in water to cover. Drain, rinse, and place the limas in a medium saucepan with fresh water to cover. Bring to a boil and reduce heat; simmer until the beans are tender, about 40 minutes to 1 hour. Drain, reserving ½ cup of the bean broth.

▶ Heat the olive oil in a large skillet over medium heat. Add the shredded brussels sprouts leaves and cook, stirring, until the greens are tender and beginning to turn golden, about 2 minutes.

Add the beans, chestnuts, brown sugar, apple cider vinegar, and the reserved bean broth. Stir together and simmer until the liquid has cooked away and everything is heated through. Season with salt and pepper to taste.

HOMEMADE SPROUTS

We like to use a mixture of clover and alfalfa seeds. Add a few radish seeds to the mix if you like a spicy kick!

Makes about 4 cups

3 tablespoons mixed seeds for sprouting
1 (1-quart) mason jar, fine cheesecloth, and rubber band

▶ Place the seeds in the mason jar and cover with water. Let them soak overnight.

▶ Cover the top of the mason jar with the cheesecloth and secure it with a rubber band. Drain off the water. Cover the seeds with some fresh cold water and swish them around briefly. Drain again.

▶ Set the mason jar on its side on a kitchen towel and cover completely with toweling (the sprouts should be kept in the dark). Rinse and drain the sprouts two times a day, more often in hotter weather. After one or two days, you should see some little sprouts starting to poke out of the seeds. After about five days, the sprouts will be about an inch long and ready to eat.

▶ Dump the sprouts out into a large mixing bowl and cover completely in cold water. Swish gently with your hands. Some of the loose seed casings will float to the surface; scoop them up with your fingers and discard them until they are mostly gone or you can't take it any more. Now lift handfuls of sprouts out of the mixing bowl and transfer them to another bowl. Unsprouted seeds and more casings will have settled to the bottom of the bowl; discard them. Place the bowl in a cool, well-lit place for a couple hours to turn green, and they are ready to eat.

▸ Store them well covered in the refrigerator and use them up quickly.

JAPANESE SPINACH

Another wonderful recipe taught to me by my aunt Julie, who learned it in the kitchen of her Japanese mother-in-law. Julie's mother-in-law reported that this was the only way she could get her sons to eat spinach when they were growing up. This is an ideal preparation for the lunch box; the spinach is ever-so-lightly blanched, not mushy, and is served cold.

Makes 3 servings

2 bunches spinach leaves (not baby spinach)

Soy sauce

Toasted sesame oil

Garlic powder

Toasted sesame seeds

▸ Wash the spinach leaves carefully to remove any sand and grit. I wash my spinach by submerging the leaves in a sink filled with cold water and agitating them gently. Lift them out of the water without draining the water first, so the dirt and sediment sinks to the bottom. Clean the sink, refill with water, and repeat until the spinach is clean. Trim off any hard pink tips on the spinach stems; otherwise leave them whole.

▸ Bring a large saucepan of water to a boil. Have a large bowl or sink filled with ice water at the ready. Dip the spinach leaves into the boiling water for just under 1 minute, just enough to cook them and leave them with a bit of crunch (or steam the spinach in a steamer basket for 1 minute, working in batches if necessary). Immediately plunge the spinach into the ice water bath to stop the cooking.

▸ Now pick up handfuls of the spinach and squeeze and knead as much water out of it as you can, transferring the squeezed spinach to a bowl. Let the spinach rest for a few minutes, then pick it up and squeeze it out again. You may want to repeat this one more time; your goal is to get as much water out of the spinach as you possibly can.

▸ Transfer the spinach to a cutting board and cut into ¾-inch pieces. Place in a bowl and sprinkle with soy sauce, 4 drops of toasted sesame oil, and garlic powder. Toss well and refrigerate until cold. Taste for seasoning and add more if desired. Sprinkle with toasted sesame seeds and serve.

LINDA'S COLLARD GREENS

My good friend from Georgia, Linda Frederick, taught me this wonderful way to prepare collard greens. Collards are an incredibly nutritious leafy green, filled with vitamin C, vitamin E, beta-carotene, calcium, and more. They are milder tasting than kale or mustard greens and are usually available year-round at the grocery store. Definitely a green worth having around!

Makes 4 servings

1 large bunch collard greens, rinsed well, hard stems removed

1 small onion, peeled and cut into quarters

A pinch of sugar

¼ cup prepared Italian dressing (or to taste)

Salt and pepper

Seasoning salt or garlic powder (optional)

- Roll the collard greens up into bundles and cut into ½-inch-wide ribbons with a sharp knife. Place the collards in a large saucepan with a tight-fitting lid. Nestle the quartered onion into the middle of the collard greens. Sprinkle with a pinch of sugar (this cuts any bitterness the greens may have) and add 1 cup of water.
- Place over high heat until the water boils, then immediately turn down the heat and cover the saucepan. Simmer the collards until they are tender when pierced with a fork, 20 to 30 minutes. Check the water level occasionally toward the end of cooking and add more water if the level gets too low.
- Drain the collards. Remove the onion or stir the onion into the collards, as you like. Toss the greens with Italian dressing, salt and pepper to taste, and garlic powder or seasoning salt as desired.

OVEN-DRIED TOMATOES

Roasting intensifies the flavor of meaty plum tomatoes and dries them out so they don't make sandwiches soggy in the lunch box.

Roast up a double batch of these on the weekend and add them to sandwiches throughout the week. They're fabulous with veggie bacon, butterhead lettuce, and vegan mayonnaise on a crusty baguette.

Makes 4 servings	6–8 medium-size plum tomatoes 1 teaspoon olive oil ¼ teaspoon kosher salt

- Preheat the oven to 250°F.
- Halve the tomatoes and place in a small mixing bowl. Toss with the olive oil and kosher salt.
- Arrange the tomatoes cut side up on a baking sheet, then roast in the oven until the tomatoes are shriveled and dry but not burnt,

about 3 hours (perhaps up to an hour more if your tomatoes are very large and juicy).

▸ Cool tomatoes completely and store in an airtight container.

PERFECT HASH BROWNS

Have you ever tried making hash browns from raw potatoes, only to have them immediately stick to your best nonstick skillet like glue? And then, after a hard-fought hash brown battle, you emerge with a sad little pile of half-burnt, half-raw potato shreds? No? Just me, huh? Well, in any case, here it is—the secret to perfect, brilliant, nonsticky hash browns!

Makes 6 hash browns	1 pound new potatoes, such as Yukon Gold 3/4 teaspoon kosher salt 3 tablespoons olive oil

▸ Peel the potatoes and shred them using a food processor fitted with a large shredding disk or a hand grater with large holes. Sprinkle the potatoes with salt and toss to coat well. Let the potatoes sit for at least 5 minutes.

▸ Then (here's the secret) take large handfuls of the potatoes and squeeze out as much liquid as you can, transferring the potatoes to a clean bowl as you go.

▸ Heat the olive oil in a large, nonstick skillet over medium-high heat. When the oil is hot (a strand of potato should sizzle when it hits the oil), pick up a handful of potato shreds, give them one last good squeeze, then drop into the oil. Repeat, making six little circular mounds of potato shreds. Press the mounds flat with your spatula and tuck the edges in to maintain an even thickness.

▸ Adjust the temperature as needed to maintain a sizzle. Cook until the bottom has turned a nice golden brown, about 8 to 10 minutes. Flip with a spatula and cook on the other side until golden brown, another 6 to 8 minutes. Drain on paper towels for a moment to remove excess oil, then place in a lunch box container and cover with foil.

POTATO "BEETLES"

Ask your kids to help you "Name That Potato." What do these potatoes look like? Are they armadillos? Roly-polies? My son says they look like beetles.

1 potato per serving	Medium-size white new potatoes
	Olive oil
	Kosher salt

▸ Line a baking sheet with parchment paper, drizzle the paper with olive oil, and set aside.

▸ Fill a medium saucepan with water, sprinkle with salt, and bring to a boil.

▸ Meanwhile, peel the new potatoes and cut in half. With a small paring knife, cut narrow slits about $1/8$ inch apart across the rounded top of each half, without going all the way through.

▸ Place the potatoes in the boiling water and boil for 5 minutes. Drain. Place them upright on the baking sheet and brush all over with olive oil. Sprinkle with kosher salt. At this point you can cover the potatoes and refrigerate until the morning, if desired.

▸ Roast the potatoes in a preheated 400°F oven until they are tender on the inside and slightly golden and crunchy on the outside, about 35 to 40 minutes.

REFRIED BLACK BEANS

It's so simple and inexpensive to prepare your own refried beans, especially if you use Slow Cooker Black Beans on page 204. Use them in burritos, tacos, tamales, or in the Layered Bean Dip on page 107.

Makes 2 cups

-----

2 tablespoons canola oil

2 cups Slow Cooker Black Beans (page 204) or 2 cups of any cooked, drained beans

1/4 cup water (or broth from cooking beans), plus more as needed

1 teaspoon cumin

1 tablespoon minced fresh cilantro

Salt

Tabasco pepper sauce

▸ In a large nonstick or cast-iron skillet, heat the oil over medium-high heat. When hot, add the beans and 1/4 cup water. Cook, stirring and smashing the beans with a wooden spoon, until the beans are a thick, coarse puree, about 10 to 15 minutes. Add more water or bean broth as needed to keep the beans from sticking and to achieve the desired consistency. Stir in the cumin and cilantro, and season with salt and Tabasco to taste.

SLOW COOKER BLACK BEANS

This is a great basic bean recipe, timed so that you will awaken to the delicious fragrance of simmering black beans in the morning, all ready to pack for lunch.

These are excellent to eat as is, served alongside greens and grains. You can also mash them into Refried Black Beans (page 203), bake them in Tennessee Corn Pone Muffins (page 218), or use them to make Sneaky Momma's Black Bean Soup (page 124). What can't these beans do?

Makes 5 cups

3 cups dried black beans

1 (4-inch) piece dried kombu seaweed (optional; kombu helps make beans more digestible)

1 onion, peeled and cut in half

2 cloves garlic, minced

2 tablespoons olive oil

¼ teaspoon liquid smoke flavoring

2 small whole dried red chile peppers

2 teaspoons kosher salt (or to taste)

▸ The morning before you want to have the beans, place the dried beans in a medium-size mixing bowl and fill the bowl with water. Set aside to soak.

▸ That evening before you go to bed, drain the beans and rinse them well. Place the beans in a medium-size (4-quart) slow cooker along with the kombu, onion, garlic, olive oil, liquid smoke, and whole dried chile peppers. Fill the slow cooker to the top with fresh water.

▸ Cover the slow cooker and cook on low overnight, or about 10 to 12 hours, until the beans are completely tender. In the morning, remove the kombu, onion, and whole dried pepper. Add salt.

TED'S ASIAN ASPARAGUS

This is it! Truly the most simple but spectacular way to enjoy the bundles of fresh, sweet asparagus that arrive at the farmers' market come springtime. This recipe was passed down to me by my stepdad, Ted, who made mountains of it for my wedding reception. The asparagus remains slightly crisp and tastes wonderful cold or at room temperature, making it ideal for the lunch box.

Makes 4 to 6 servings

2 pounds fresh asparagus, washed and trimmed

2 tablespoons peanut oil

1 tablespoon soy sauce

Toasted sesame seeds

▸ Cut each asparagus spear into three 1½- to 2-inch pieces, separating out the tips and setting them aside. Have a bowl of ice water ready.

▸ Bring a small saucepan of salted water to a boil and add the cut asparagus stalks. Boil until the asparagus is slightly tender but still crisp, about 2 to 3 minutes. Remove the asparagus from the water with a slotted spoon and immediately plunge it into ice water to stop cooking.

▸ Repeat the process with the asparagus tips, boiling them for about 1 minute then plunging them into the ice water. Drain the stalks and tips and place them in a serving bowl.

▸ Whisk together the peanut oil and soy sauce and pour over the asparagus, tossing gently. Top with toasted sesame seeds.

BREADS AND MUFFINS

Quick Breads

BLACKSTRAP GINGERBREAD WITH LEMON SAUCE TOPPING

Hands down, this is the best gingerbread we have ever had. This recipe is from the charming booklet *The Happy Lunchbox* by my wonderful friend Renee Pottle, who was kind enough to let me share it here.

Because this gingerbread has no sweetener besides molasses, using all blackstrap might make it a little strong for your taste. You can use sweet molasses instead or a combination of both.

We have an old family tradition of always serving gingerbread with lemon sauce, so I've added one here. Store the sauce in a separate container to pour over the gingerbread just before eating.

Makes 9 large servings	1 3/4 cups all-purpose flour
	1/4 cup potato flour
	1/2 cup whole wheat flour
	1 1/2 teaspoons baking soda

1 teaspoon cinnamon

1 teaspoon ginger

½ teaspoon allspice

A pinch of salt

1 cup molasses

½ cup canola oil

1 cup hot water

¼ cup candied ginger (optional)

▸ Preheat oven to 350°F. In an 8 x 8-inch baking dish, mix together the flours, baking soda, cinnamon, ginger, allspice, and salt with a fork.

▸ Add molasses, canola oil, and water. Mix well, using the fork to break up all lumps. Stir in the candied ginger, if using.

▸ Bake for 35 to 40 minutes (it took 45 minutes in my oven) or until a wooden pick inserted in the middle comes out clean.

▸ Set the pan on a wire rack to cool.

LEMON SAUCE

A sweet sauce perfect for topping Blackstrap Gingerbread or spooning onto Blueberry Lemon Mini Scones (page 209).

Makes about
1 cup

½ cup sugar

1 tablespoon cornstarch

1 cup water

⅛ cup nonhydrogenated margarine

1 tablespoon freshly squeezed lemon juice

Zest of one lemon

- Whisk sugar and cornstarch together in a small saucepan. Gradually stir in water and heat over medium-high heat until boiling, stirring constantly with a wooden spoon. Boil for 2 minutes, until sugar has dissolved and the sauce has thickened.
- Remove from heat and stir in the margarine, lemon juice, and zest. Serve immediately or refrigerate several hours or overnight; the sauce will thicken more as it cools.

BLUEBERRY LEMON MINI SCONES

This recipe was a gift from baker-genius Tina Stephenson at Badger Canyon Herb & Tea in Kennewick, Washington. Tina makes a batch of vegan cookies or scones every Friday, and boy, if you don't get there before noon, they are gone. Luckily, she was nice enough to share the secret to her scone success with me. Now when I snooze and lose, I can go home and whip up a batch of my very own.

Makes 12
mini scones

1 cup all-purpose flour

1 cup whole wheat pastry flour

¼ cup sugar

2 teaspoons baking powder

½ teaspoon baking soda

½ teaspoon kosher salt

¼ cup nonhydrogenated margarine

½ cup plain, unsweetened soymilk

¾ cup fresh or thawed frozen blueberries, rinsed and drained

Zest of one lemon

Extra soymilk and sugar for topping

- Preheat the oven to 400°F. Line a baking sheet with parchment paper and spray with nonstick spray. Set aside.
- Sift together the flours, sugar, baking powder, baking soda, and salt. Add the margarine and cut into the flour mixture using a pastry cutter or your fingers, until the mixture resembles a coarse, crumbly meal.
- Add the soymilk, blueberries, and zest. Mix well with a wooden spoon or your hands until the mixture comes together to form a dough. You may need to add an extra tablespoon of soymilk if the mixture is too dry.
- Turn the dough out onto a lightly floured work surface. Divide the dough in half and form each half into a flat round, about ¾ inch thick. Cut each round into six equal wedges.
- Arrange the scones on the baking sheet. Brush the tops with a bit of soymilk and sprinkle with sugar. Bake for 15 to 18 minutes, until the edges and bottom are golden. Place scones on a wire rack to cool.

VARIATION: Cherry Almond Mini Scones: Follow directions above, but replace the blueberries with ¾ cup fresh or thawed frozen sweet or pie cherries, pitted and coarsely chopped. Replace the lemon zest with 1 teaspoon almond extract.

EASY PIECRUST

This is a simple, satisfying, no-frills piecrust. Master it, and you will have dozens of delicious lunchtime possibilities at your fingertips. Start with Spanish Empanadas (page 175), Cornish Pasties (page 153), or Aloo Samosas (page 143). Then use your imagination and wrap mushrooms, tofu, or any of your favorite vegetables in light, flaky pastry. Heck, you could even bake a pie!

Makes 1 (9-inch) pie shell

---
2 cups all-purpose flour (or half white, half whole wheat pastry flour)

1 teaspoon kosher salt

2/3 cup nonhydrogenated shortening

5–7 tablespoons ice water, as needed

▸ Have a cup of ice water and a tablespoon ready.

▸ Sift or whisk together the flour and salt in a mixing bowl. Dot the top of the flour mixture with tablespoons of the shortening. Cut the shortening into the flour with a pastry cutter or by tossing and rubbing the flour and shortening together with your hands or fingers. Keep at it until the mixture resembles coarse meal and all visible lumps of shortening are gone.

▸ Lightly drizzle in the water a tablespoon at a time, stirring with a wooden spoon or your fingers, until you can bring the dough together in a ball. Add a few extra drops if the dough is still crumbly. Shape the dough into a ball, then proceed with your recipe.

▸ If it's a hot day, you may wish to refrigerate the dough for 15 minutes before rolling and shaping.

FULL MEAL MUFFINS

When I was working on the first edition of *Vegan Lunch Box*, I came up with the idea of including a "Full Meal Muffin" recipe that would serve as a convenient, portable, inconspicuous lunch for older kids and teens that included fruits and vegetables. At the time I also wanted to include protein powder for a protein boost, but I was never satisfied with the texture and taste of the muffins with added powder.

After several unsuccessful attempts I decided to bag the muffin idea, but several distraught readers later e-mailed, asking what had happened to it. So I dusted off my notes, kicked out the protein powder, and here it is! Even without the extra protein this is a nutritious main course at lunchtime: each muffin is filled with whole grains, banana, zucchini, iron- and calcium-rich blackstrap molasses, and omega–3-rich walnuts. These muffins also contain no added sugar, salt, oil, soy, or wheat.

Makes 12 muffins

1 cup whole spelt flour

1 cup barley flour (or use 1 cup white and 1 cup whole wheat flour in place of spelt and barley if you prefer)

1 teaspoon cinnamon

2 teaspoons baking powder

1 teaspoon baking soda

2 ripe bananas, peeled

3 tablespoons blackstrap molasses

1/2 cup apple juice, plus more as needed

2 teaspoons apple cider vinegar

1 zucchini, finely grated (about 1 1/2 cups)

1/2 cup finely chopped or ground walnuts

1/2 cup currants or raisins (optional, they add a touch of sweetness)

- Preheat the oven to 375°F. Line a muffin tin with paper liners and spray with nonstick spray and set aside.
- Combine both flours, cinnamon, baking powder, and baking soda in a mixing bowl and whisk together.
- Place the bananas, blackstrap molasses, apple juice, and apple cider vinegar in a blender and blend until smooth. Mix the wet and dry ingredients together, then fold in the zucchini, walnuts, and currants or raisins, if using. Use a bit more apple juice if needed to wet all the flour.
- Divide the mixture evenly into the twelve lined muffin cups and bake for 20 minutes or until the top springs back to the touch. Remove muffins from the pan and cool on a wire rack.
- Store in an airtight container or freeze in individual freezer bags to pull out and put into lunches as needed.

PEANUT BUTTER AND JELLY MUFFINS

If you don't have a piping bag, not to worry: simply cut open the muffin and spread it with a liberal layer of jam. These muffins are wheat-free.

Makes 12 muffins

1 1/2 cups barley flour

1/2 cup oat bran (or oat flour)

2 1/2 teaspoons baking powder

1/4 teaspoon kosher salt

1/2 cup applesauce

3/4 cup natural creamy peanut butter

1/4 cup maple syrup

1 cup plain soymilk

3 tablespoons finely chopped unsalted peanuts

About 12 tablespoons fruit spread,
   jam, or jelly

- Preheat the oven to 375°F. Line a muffin tin with paper liners or spray with nonstick spray. Set aside.
- In a large mixing bowl, whisk together the barley flour, oat bran, baking powder, and salt. In another bowl, mix together the applesauce, peanut butter, maple syrup, and soymilk. Add the wet ingredients to the dry ingredients, mixing until well combined.
- Spoon the batter evenly into twelve muffin cups. Sprinkle the tops with peanuts and bake for 20 to 25 minutes, until a toothpick inserted in the center comes out clean. Place the muffins on a wire rack to cool completely.
- When cool, use a piping bag with a sharp metal star tip to push into the top of each muffin and pipe a tablespoon of jam through into the center.

PUMPKIN CAROB CHIP MUFFINS

Muffins are a great way to make orange vegetables attractive to a child who might otherwise dislike them. Filled with nutritious whole wheat, flaxseed, pumpkin, and nuts, they are soy-free for those with soy allergies. Carob chips taste just right here, but feel free to substitute vegan chocolate chips if you prefer.

Makes 12 muffins

1 cup plain canned pumpkin (not pumpkin pie filling) or pureed butternut squash

$1/3$ cup water

$1/3$ cup canola oil

2 tablespoons ground flaxseed

1 teaspoon vanilla

$1 2/3$ cups whole wheat pastry flour

$1 1/3$ cups sugar

1 teaspoon baking powder

½ teaspoon baking soda
½ teaspoon kosher salt
½ teaspoon cinnamon
¼ teaspoon nutmeg
⅓ cup vegan carob chips
½ cup pecans, chopped
Perfect Cinnamon-Sugar (see below)

▶ Preheat the oven to 350°F. Spray a nonstick muffin tin with non-stick spray or line the tin with paper muffin cups and spray the cups with nonstick spray. Set aside.

▶ Put the pumpkin, water, canola oil, flaxseed, and vanilla in a blender and process on high for at least 1 minute, until light in color and well blended. Set aside.

▶ In a large mixing bowl, whisk together the pastry flour, sugar, baking powder, baking soda, salt, cinnamon, and nutmeg. Add the pumpkin mixture and mix with a wooden spoon or large spatula until well blended. Fold in the carob chips and pecans.

▶ Spoon the batter into the muffin tin, distributing evenly to make twelve muffins. Sprinkle the top of each muffin with some Perfect Cinnamon-Sugar.

▶ Bake for 30 to 35 minutes, until a cake tester or toothpick inserted into the center of a muffin comes out clean. Let cool for 5 minutes in the pan, then use a spatula to gently lift each muffin from the muffin tin. Finish cooling on a wire rack.

Perfect Cinnamon-Sugar

▶ Whisk together ¾ cup sugar with 2 teaspoons ground cinnamon and store in a sugar shaker. Use as a sweet sprinkle on porridge, toast, or soy yogurt.

SPELT BISCUITS

These wheat-free biscuits come together in a flash in the food processor.

Makes 14 biscuits

1 cup plain soymilk

2 teaspoons apple cider vinegar

1 3/4 cups white spelt flour

3/4 cup whole spelt flour

2 teaspoons baking powder

1/2 teaspoon baking soda

1/2 teaspoon kosher salt

6 tablespoons nonhydrogenated margarine
    or shortening

▸ Preheat oven to 450°F. Line a baking sheet with parchment paper and spray with nonstick spray. Set aside.

▸ In a 2-cup liquid measuring cup or small bowl, combine the soymilk and apple cider vinegar. The mixture will thicken slightly and curdle—now you have soy "buttermilk"! Set aside.

▸ In the bowl of a food processor fitted with the S blade, combine the spelt flours, baking powder, baking soda, and salt. Pulse briefly to combine. Take the lid off the food processor and drop the margarine by tablespoonfuls evenly over the surface of the flour mixture. Pulse several times until the margarine has worked itself into the flour mixture and no large lumps remain.

▸ Add the soy "buttermilk" and run the food processor just enough to form a dough. Scrape the dough out onto a lightly floured countertop or kneading board.

▸ Pat the dough into a circle about 1 inch thick. Cut the dough into rounds using a 2½-inch biscuit cutter or the rim of a glass; dip the cutter in flour in between cuts to prevent sticking.

▸ Place the biscuits on the prepared baking sheet and bake until light brown, about 12 minutes.

VARIATION: If you'd like to make biscuits using regular white flour, substitute 2 cups all-purpose flour for both the spelt flours.

> ## "CAN I HELP?"
>
> I still remember standing on a stool in my grandfather's kitchen helping him cut out biscuits with a round metal cutter. Perhaps that's when my love of cooking began! Make fun memories with your children, letting them pat down the dough and cut out these biscuits. You can even use the leftover dough scraps to form smiling faces or designs on the biscuit tops.

SWEET CORNBREAD

This is the kind of sweet, tender cornbread that I prefer, the kind my mother would insist is properly referred to as "johnnycake." Bread or cake, this recipe is so easy, so tasty, and no, it's not crumbly! It was shared by Amy Nylund and Candace d'Obrenovic, members of Vegetarian Network of Austin, Texas, and immediately became our favorite cornbread of all time. Thanks, Amy and Candace!

Makes one
9 x 9-inch pan

$2/3$ cup maple syrup

$1/3$ cup canola oil

1 cup plain soymilk

1 cup whole wheat flour

1 cup fine organic cornmeal

1 tablespoon baking powder

1 teaspoon kosher salt

- Preheat the oven to 350°F. Spray a 9 x 9-inch baking pan with nonstick spray and set aside.
- In a small mixing bowl, combine the maple syrup, canola oil, and soymilk. In another bowl, whisk together the whole wheat flour, cornmeal, baking powder, and salt. Mix wet and dry mixtures together and pour the batter into the prepared pan. Bake for 35 minutes, or until a toothpick or cake tester comes out clean.

VARIATION: For individual-sized cornbreads just right for the lunch box, try baking the cornbread in muffin cups or mini loaf pans for about 25 minutes.

VARIATION: Vegan Corn Dogs! Visit the Vegan Lunch Box and find out how to transform this Sweet Cornbread into Vegan Corn Dogs: veganlunchbox.blogspot.com/2006/03/corn-dog.html.

TENNESSEE CORN PONE MUFFINS

Traditional Tennessee Corn Pone consists of a layer of cornbread baked over a bed of flavorful beans. These cornmeal muffins are made on the same principle but with the beans spooned into the batter on top, to make them easier to eat out of hand at lunchtime. They are gluten-free and a great source of heart-healthy omega–3 fats from flax.

Makes 12 muffins

1 cup plain soymilk
2 teaspoons apple cider vinegar
4 tablespoons ground flaxseed
1 cup fine organic cornmeal
1 teaspoon baking soda
1/2 teaspoon kosher salt

1 cup Slow Cooker Black Beans (page 204) or
other well-seasoned cooked beans, drained
Nutritional yeast flakes (optional)

▸ Preheat the oven to 400°F. Spray a nonstick muffin tin with non-stick spray or line the tin with paper muffin cups and spray the cups with nonstick spray. Set aside.
▸ In a 2-cup liquid measuring cup or small mixing bowl, whisk the soymilk, apple cider vinegar, and ground flaxseed together. Set aside.
▸ In a medium-size mixing bowl, whisk together the cornmeal, baking soda, and salt. Pour the soymilk mixture into the cornmeal mixture and stir together until well combined.
▸ Divide the cornmeal mixture evenly among the twelve muffin cups. Drain any excess liquid off the beans (they should be slightly juicy but not too wet). Top each muffin with a large spoonful of beans. Sprinkle each muffin with nutritional yeast flakes if desired.
▸ Bake the muffins for about 15 minutes, until set and golden brown around the edges. Let the muffins cool in the tin for about 5 to 10 minutes, then carefully remove the muffins using a spatula and place them on a wire rack to cool completely.

Yeast Breads

BLUE RIBBON BREAD

This is my favorite bread recipe, and the one I enter every year in our local county fair. It always gets a blue ribbon (and once got Best of Show). I hope it wins awards at your table, too!

This recipe makes a lot of bread. I figure if I'm making bread I might as well make enough to last a while (because I know the first loaf is going to be gone an hour after it leaves the oven). It freezes well, too.

The leftover cooked grains called for here can be practically anything; I have had excellent results using cooked steel-cut oats, polenta, brown or white rice, quinoa, or a combination. If the cooked grains are particularly wet, you may need to add more flour.

Makes three (8.5 x 3.5-inch) loaves or two loaves and one 9 x 9-inch pan of dinner rolls

---
2 cups warm water (110°F)

2 scant tablespoons (2 packages) active dry yeast

½ cup canola oil

½ cup maple syrup

1 tablespoon kosher salt

2 cups leftover cooked grains (see note above), room temperature

3 cups whole wheat flour

4–5 cups white bread flour

- Pour the warm water into a very large mixing bowl. Sprinkle the yeast over the warm water and stir well. Let the mixture sit for 5 minutes to dissolve the yeast.
- Add the canola oil, maple syrup, kosher salt, cooked grains, and whole wheat flour to the yeast water, stirring vigorously. Beat well with a large wooden spoon. This mixture is called the "sponge" and should be wetter and softer than bread dough. Cover with plastic wrap and let the sponge rise in a warm, draft-free place for 1½ hours.
- Stir the sponge down and add 3 cups of the white bread flour, stirring in about ½ cup at a time until the mixture is firm enough to knead by hand. Turn the dough out onto a well-floured counter or pastry board and knead vigorously. Sprinkle more flour on your hands and the work surface as you knead to keep the dough from sticking. You will need to add about 1½ cups more white bread flour in this way, more if the leftover grains you used were particularly moist. Knead for 20 minutes, until the dough is smooth and develops an inner firmness and a springy quality.
- Shape the dough into a round and place it in a very large, well-oiled mixing bowl (the largest you've got—it gets crazy big), turning the round so the top of the dough gets coated with some of the oil. Cover with plastic and let rise in a warm, draft-free place until doubled in bulk, about 1 hour.
- Punch the dough down and turn out onto a lightly floured work surface. Flatten out the dough with your hands, pressing out any air bubbles. Cut the dough into three equal pieces. Shape into three loaves and place in three 8.5 x 3.5-inch loaf pans that have been sprayed with nonstick spray. Or shape into two loaves and divide the rest of the dough into nine pieces; shape each piece into a round and space them evenly apart in a 9 x 9-inch baking pan that has been sprayed with nonstick spray. Spray or brush the

tops of the bread gently with olive oil, cover lightly with plastic wrap, and let the bread rise one last time.

▸ During the final rise preheat the oven to 375°F. When the loaves and rolls have risen until not quite doubled, about 25 minutes, place in the oven. Bake until golden and hollow sounding when given a gentle thump, about 20 to 25 minutes for rolls, 35 to 40 minutes for bread. Rotate the pans once during baking to ensure even baking.

▸ Remove the bread and rolls from the pans immediately and cool on a wire rack.

CROISSANTS

This is my veganized, whole wheat version of a recipe from *The Fannie Farmer Baking Book*. My husband called these "uncommonly good" and promised to gain weight if I would make them more often.

Slice the croissants in half and fill them with vegan ham deli slices and a slice of vegan cheese for classic Ham and Cheese Croissants.

Makes 16 croissants

1 ¼ cups plain soymilk, warmed

1 tablespoon sugar

2 ¼ teaspoons (1 package) active dry yeast

1 ½ cups all-purpose flour, plus more
   as needed

1 cup whole wheat flour (preferably
   graham flour)

1 ¼ teaspoons kosher salt

¾ cup nonhydrogenated margarine, cold

- Put the soymilk into a large mixing bowl, add the sugar and yeast, and whisk to dissolve. Let the yeast mixture sit for a few minutes until foamy.
- Mix together the flour, whole wheat flour, and salt. Add the flour mixture to the yeast mixture and stir until a sticky dough forms. Turn the dough out onto a liberally floured surface and knead for a few strokes, just long enough to form a smooth dough. Add flour as needed.
- Roll the dough with a floured rolling pin into a 9 x 14-inch rectangle.
- Put the margarine between two sheets of wax paper and roll out into a 6 x 8-inch rectangle. Peel off the wax paper and place the margarine on the bottom half of the dough. Fold the bottom, sides, and top half over the margarine, encasing the margarine completely. Sprinkle the dough with flour, cover with plastic or place in a plastic bag, and refrigerate for 45 minutes.
- *First turn*: place the dough on a liberally floured work surface and roll out with a floured rolling pin using firm, smooth strokes. Roll out to 9 x 14 inches, then fold the bottom and top halves in toward the center (like folding up a letter). Sprinkle with flour, cover with plastic again, and refrigerate for 45 minutes.
- *Second turn*: repeat as above, refrigerating for 45 minutes.
- *Third turn*: repeat as above, refrigerating for 45 minutes.
- *Shape the croissants*: Line a baking sheet with parchment paper, spray with nonstick spray, and set aside. Roll the dough out on a well-floured surface to about 10 x 20 inches. Cut the rectangle in half lengthwise, then cut into eight squares. Cut each square in half diagonally to form sixteen triangles.
- Pull the top triangle point out a little to lengthen, then start at the bottom of the triangle and roll it up tightly. Tuck the tip under and curve the edges in to form a croissant shape; press down lightly on the top to help the croissant hold its shape. Repeat

with the remaining croissants, placing them on the baking sheet about 2 inches apart. Spray the croissants with nonstick spray, cover lightly with plastic wrap, and let rise in a warm place for about 1½ hours, until light and puffy.

▸ Meanwhile, preheat the oven to 425°F.

▸ Bake the croissants for 10 minutes, then reduce the heat to 375°F and bake for an additional 10 minutes, or until golden brown. If they are browning too quickly on the bottom, try insulating them by putting another baking pan underneath the croissant pan.

▸ Cool on a wire rack.

EASY WHOLE-GRAIN PIZZA DOUGH

This quick and tasty dough is used to make the Broccoli Calzones (page 147) and the Mini Vegan Pizzas on page 160. You can make the dough quickly in a food processor. If you don't have a food processor, you can follow the instructions for Pizza Shop Breadsticks on page 227 to mix and knead the dough by hand.

Makes enough dough for 8 calzones or 8 mini pizzas

1½ cups warm water (110°F)
2¼ teaspoons (1 package) active dry yeast
3 cups all-purpose flour
¾ cup whole wheat flour
¼ cup finely ground cornmeal
1½ teaspoons kosher salt
2 tablespoons extra virgin olive oil

▸ In a small bowl, sprinkle the yeast in the warm water and stir well to dissolve. Set the yeast aside for about 5 minutes to bloom.

- Meanwhile, place the flours, cornmeal, and salt together in the bowl of a food processor fitted with the S blade. Pulse well to combine.
- With the food processor running, slowing drizzle the yeast mixture into the feed tube. Stop when the dough forms a ball. Pour in the olive oil and pulse two or three times to combine.
- Turn the dough onto a lightly floured surface and knead briefly, just long enough to incorporate any scraps from the food processor and make a smooth dough. Proceed with your calzone or pizza recipe.

ETHIOPIAN INJERA BREAD

These soft, spongy flatbreads are made with teff flour. Teff is the world's tiniest cultivated grain and one of the most nutritious. Injera batter is traditionally left at room temperature for several days to ferment and develop a sourdoughlike tang. This batter uses yeast and a quick rise instead and has less of a sour taste. Teff flour can be found at natural food stores.

Makes about
6 to 7 large injera
(serves 4)

---

2 cups warm water (110°F)

1 teaspoon sugar

1 teaspoon active dry yeast

1 cup teff flour

1 cup all-purpose flour

½ teaspoon kosher salt

Canola oil for cooking

- In a medium-size mixing bowl, dissolve the sugar and yeast in the warm water. Let the yeast mixture sit for about 5 minutes to allow the yeast to dissolve and become active.

▸ Slowly add the teff flour, all-purpose flour, and salt to the yeast mixture, whisking constantly. Whisk the batter vigorously for 2 minutes. Cover with plastic wrap and let rise in a warm place for 1 hour. At this point, the batter can be refrigerated for several hours or overnight.

▸ Heat a 10-inch, well-seasoned cast-iron or nonstick skillet over medium heat. When the skillet is hot, drizzle with a small amount of oil and spread the oil evenly over the surface of the skillet. Stir the batter, then pour ½ cup of it on the hot skillet. Quickly tilt the pan to evenly distribute the batter in a large circle.

▸ Cover the pan with a lid and cook for 2 minutes, then remove the lid (lift quickly to avoid dropping condensed drops of moisture onto the injera and wipe the inner lid dry between injera). Cook for another few seconds, until the top surface is dry and springs back to the touch. The top should be covered with bubbles and the bottom should be lightly golden (lower the heat if the bottom is browning too quickly). Run a spatula around the edges of the injera to help release it from the pan, then lift the injera from the skillet with the spatula and place it on a wire rack to cool (injera is only cooked on one side). Repeat with the remaining batter. When the injera have cooled, stack them on a serving plate. Injera are served warm or at room temperature.

▸ To serve, place one injera on a plate and top with Split Pea Alecha (page 126) and/or Mixed Vegetable Wat (page 120). Tear off pieces to scoop up bits of stew and pop them in your mouth.

▸ To pack in a lunch box, roll up the injera bread while it's still a bit warm, then slice into bite-size pieces. Pack along with both stews for dipping.

PIZZA SHOP BREADSTICKS

These breadsticks are made with high-protein semolina flour. Semolina flour is made from durum wheat (the same wheat used to make many pastas). It is rough and granular and light yellow in color. It is available at some health food stores and Italian markets. Feel free to substitute whole wheat flour if you can't find semolina.

You will need a spice grinder or strong blender (see page 116) to make the "cheesy" breadstick topping.

Makes 36 breadsticks

3/4 cup warm water (110°F)

1/2 teaspoon sugar

1 teaspoon active dry yeast

1 cup all-purpose flour or white bread flour

1 cup semolina flour, plus more for the baking sheets

2 tablespoons raw wheat germ

1/2 teaspoon kosher salt

1 tablespoon extra virgin olive oil, plus more for brushing

1/4 cup raw sesame seeds

1/8 cup nutritional yeast flakes

1/2 teaspoon salt (or to taste)

1/8 teaspoon garlic granules

1/8 teaspoon freshly ground black pepper

▶ In a mug or liquid measuring cup, dissolve the sugar and yeast in the warm water. Let the yeast mixture sit for about 5 minutes to dissolve and become active (the yeast should start to foam or bubble slightly). Meanwhile, combine the flour, semolina flour, wheat germ, and kosher salt in a medium-size mixing bowl.

- Add the yeast mixture and olive oil and stir well with a wooden spoon until a dough forms. Turn the dough out onto a clean, flat work surface and knead for about 10 minutes, until the dough is smooth and firm. Sprinkle your work surface with a bit of flour, if necessary, to keep the dough from sticking.

- Place the dough in a mixing bowl that has been brushed or sprayed with olive oil. Turn the dough over to coat the top with oil. Cover the bowl with plastic wrap and a clean kitchen towel. Let the dough rise in a warm, draft-free place for 40 minutes.

- Meanwhile, line two baking sheets with parchment paper and sprinkle with a bit of semolina flour (or use cornmeal if not using semolina). Set aside.

- Preheat the oven to 375°F and prepare the topping: grind the sesame seeds in a spice grinder until they resemble a coarse meal. Pour the sesame seeds into a small dish and stir in the nutritional yeast, salt, garlic granules, and pepper to taste.

- Turn the dough out onto a flat work surface that has been sprinkled with flour. Use a rolling pin to roll the dough into a 14 x 10-inch rectangle. Brush the entire top surface with olive oil. Sprinkle liberally and evenly with the sesame seed topping. Use your fingers to gently press the topping into the dough.

- Use a pizza wheel or sharp knife to cut the dough into eighteen 3/4-inch-wide strips. Then cut all the strips in half, so that you have thirty-six 5-inch long breadsticks. Pick up each breadstick and twist it several times, then place breadsticks about 1 inch apart on the baking sheet. Press the ends down firmly onto the baking sheet to keep them from untwisting.

- At this point, the breadsticks may be covered with plastic wrap and refrigerated several hours or overnight. Bake for 12 to 15 minutes, or until golden. Serve with tomato sauce for dipping.

PUMPKIN ANADAMA ROLLS

Anadama Bread is a fine old American recipe with a colorful history. Legend has it that it was first made by a man whose wife, Anna, left him with nothing but some cornmeal mush to his name. He made it into bread, all the while muttering, "Anna, damn her!" You may or may not want to share that story with your child. . . .

The recipe starts with a homemade cornmeal mush, which has been a staple food in America since ancient times. I have added some pumpkin to my recipe, to give the bread a lovely golden color, and to add another interesting native food to the menu.

Makes 12 rolls	1 ½ cups plain soymilk
	¼ cup cornmeal
	2 tablespoons dark molasses
	2 tablespoons nonhydrogenated margarine
	1 teaspoon kosher salt
	½ cup plain canned pumpkin (not pumpkin pie filling) or pureed butternut squash
	2 ¼ teaspoons (1 package) active dry yeast
	1 cup whole wheat flour
	2 cups all-purpose flour or white bread flour, plus more as needed

▸ Warm ¾ cup of the soymilk in a small saucepan. When the soymilk is almost boiling, sprinkle in the cornmeal, whisking constantly. Cook, stirring, for 5 minutes, until the cornmeal has thickened. Set aside to cool to room temperature.

▸ Warm the remaining ¾ cup soymilk in a small saucepan along with the molasses, margarine, salt, and pumpkin. Heat until the mixture is warm to the touch (110°F). Pour the mixture into a mixing bowl. Sprinkle with the active dry yeast, stir, and let stand for about 5 minutes to dissolve and become active; the yeast should start to foam or bubble slightly.

- Meanwhile, whisk together the whole wheat and white flour. Lightly oil a mixing bowl and set aside. Line a baking sheet with parchment paper, spray with nonstick spray, and set aside.
- When the yeast has dissolved, add the cooled cornmeal mush and the flour. Beat with a wooden spoon or mix well with your hands until a dough forms and pulls away from the sides of the bowl. Turn out onto a lightly floured work surface. Knead until the dough is smooth and elastic, about 10 minutes, adding up to a cup of white flour as needed to keep the dough from sticking.
- Put the dough into the oiled bowl, turning it to coat it with oil. Cover with plastic wrap and let it rise until it has doubled in bulk, about 30 minutes.
- Turn out the dough onto a lightly floured surface and press out the air bubbles. Divide the dough into twelve equal pieces, and shape each piece into a smooth, round ball. Place the rolls 1 inch apart on the baking sheet, spray lightly with olive oil, and cover lightly with plastic wrap. Let rise for 25 minutes, preheating the oven to 375°F in the last ten minutes of rising.
- Remove the plastic wrap and bake the rolls for 18 to 20 minutes, until lightly browned. Cool the rolls on a wire rack.

DESSERTS

SWEETS AND TREATS

Some of the desserts you'll find in this cookbook are the kind of super-healthy goodies that make a parent jump for joy when their kids ask for seconds or thirds. For example, Cherry Chip Brownies (page 236) and Fruit and Nut Bars (page 237) are low in refined sugar and rich in whole grains, dried fruit, and heart-healthy nuts.

Other desserts, like the following cupcakes, are sugary, decadent concoctions I save for extra-special occasions, like birthdays. These are the treats I whip up for parties and for impressing the omnivores.

You'll notice I also call for various store-bought cookies and sweets in my lunch menus. I wanted to give you an idea of how easy it is to find vegan goodies that kids can feel right at home eating alongside their omni peers in the cafeteria. You may or may not want to include a little sugary treat in the lunch box each day, depending on your family's health and sugar sensitivity.

Whatever your take on dessert, don't overdo it! Once, during our first weeks of packed lunches, I packed James four crème-filled cookies. I was aghast when he came home, and I discovered most of his lunch entirely uneaten. "I ate the cookies first," he reported, "and then I was full." Someone reading this story on my blog shared this tip: "My mom used to say 'One cookie for each hand.' We never got more than two cookies a day." I've taken that as my rule of thumb, and it has held me in good stead ever since.

Cookies and Bars

BACK-TO-SCHOOL CHOCOLATE CHIP COOKIES

During those fleeting final days of summer, get the kids together in the kitchen to bake these easy chocolate chip cookies. They freeze brilliantly; after they have cooled, I place sets of two or three into small resealable plastic bags in the freezer to pull out and toss in lunch boxes on busy mornings. Let's just hope you can get some in the freezer before they disappear!

Makes 4 dozen cookies

2 $\frac{1}{4}$ cups whole wheat pastry flour (or barley flour)

$\frac{3}{4}$ teaspoon baking soda

$\frac{1}{4}$ teaspoon kosher salt

1 cup nonhydrogenated margarine, at room temperature

$\frac{3}{4}$ cup packed golden brown sugar

$\frac{3}{4}$ cup sugar

$\frac{3}{4}$ cup soft silken tofu, drained

1 $\frac{1}{2}$ teaspoons vanilla

1 cup vegan chocolate chips

$\frac{3}{4}$ cup chopped walnuts or pecans

▸ Preheat the oven to 375°F. Line two baking sheets with parchment paper, spray with nonstick spray, and set aside.

- In a medium mixing bowl, whisk together the flour, baking soda, and salt. Set aside.
- In another mixing bowl, combine the margarine, sugars, tofu, and vanilla. Beat with a handheld mixer until light and fluffy, stopping to scrape down the sides of the bowl. Add the dry ingredients and beat well. Fold in the chocolate chips and nuts with a spatula.
- Using a 1-ounce cookie scoop or a large spoon, place scoops of cookie dough on the baking sheets about 3 inches apart. Bake until golden brown around the edges, about 12 minutes.
- Using a spatula, transfer the cookies from the baking sheet to a wire rack to cool completely. Store in an airtight container.
- Note: if it's a warm day, place the bowl of cookie dough in the refrigerator between batches so the dough doesn't get all melty (melty dough equals thin, flat cookies).

BANANA OATMEAL COOKIES

Cookies without wheat, sugar, oil, or salt? You betcha! You'll need a good, strong blender like a Vita-Mix (see page 116) to blend the oats into a fine flour; otherwise, purchase oat flour at the health food store.

Makes about 24 cookies

2 cups oats

$3/4$ teaspoon baking soda

1 teaspoon cinnamon

4 medium-size overripe bananas, peeled

$1/4$ cup sunflower seeds

$1/4$ cup chopped dates

- Preheat the oven to 350°F. Line a baking sheet with parchment paper and spray with nonstick spray. Set aside.

- Use a good blender to blend the oats into fine flour. Pour the oat flour into a mixing bowl and add the baking soda and cinnamon.
- Put the bananas into the blender and blend until completely smooth. Add to the oat mixture along with the sunflower seeds and dates and mix until well combined.
- Use a 1-ounce cookie scoop to place spoonfuls of the cookie dough on the baking sheet.
- Bake for 12 minutes. Cool cookies on a wire rack and store in an airtight container in the refrigerator.

CASHEW CRISPY SQUARES

Marshmallow rice squares are a perennial kid's favorite. Unfortunately, the mainstream variety contains butter and animal gelatin (in the marshmallows). Lucky for us, this vegan version is just as crispy, sweet, and gooey!

These squares are also the perfect dessert for those children who can't have wheat, gluten, or soy. Fold in some vegan chocolate chips for an extra-decadent treat.

Makes 12 large squares

5 cups organic brown rice crisps cereal
   (I recommend Barbara's Bakery brand)
1 cup sugar
1/2 cup organic light corn syrup
1/4 cup plain rice milk
6 tablespoons creamy unsalted cashew butter
1/2 cup vegan chocolate chips or dried
   blueberries (optional)

- Spray a 9 x 9-inch baking pan with nonstick spray and set aside. Put the rice cereal in a large mixing bowl and set aside.

- In a small saucepan, combine the sugar, corn syrup, and rice milk. Heat over medium-high heat, stirring constantly, until the mixture starts boiling. At this point, stop stirring and let the mixture boil, without stirring, for 6 minutes (in candy making this is called the "soft-ball stage"). Watch it carefully; the mixture should maintain a rolling, foamy boil. If it starts to rise up and overflow from the pan, quickly remove the pan from heat, lower the heat a bit, then return the pan to the burner.
- Meanwhile, measure out the 6 tablespoons of cashew butter into a small bowl so it's ready to go.
- After 6 minutes, remove the pan from the heat and immediately add the cashew butter. Stir until well combined, then quickly drizzle the mixture over the rice, stirring with a large spatula until evenly distributed. If using chocolate chips or dried blueberries, fold them in.
- Press the rice mixture evenly into the 9 x 9-inch pan. Let cool completely, then cut into squares. Store in an airtight container.

CHERRY CHIP BROWNIES

These are moist, dense, and chewy—just like brownies ought to be—but without the sugar-induced coma of a regular brownie. They are a treat you can feel good about serving often, filled as they are with wholesome dried fruit and omega–3-rich walnuts.

I have the cutest picture of James eating these (without the nuts) in his high chair as a toddler. He is covered with carob all the way up to his ears and is smiling contentedly. Now I feed them to my little two-year-old niece, Summer Irene, who enjoys them just as much as her big cousin.

Makes one
9 x 9-inch pan,
about 16 brownies

$^1/_2$ cup packed pitted dates

$^1/_2$ cup packed pitted dried plums

1 cup barley flour

1 cup brown rice flour

$^1/_3$ cup carob powder (or cocoa powder)

1 $^1/_2$ teaspoons baking powder

$^1/_2$ teaspoon kosher salt

$^2/_3$ cup maple syrup

$^1/_4$ cup canola oil

1 teaspoon vanilla

$^3/_4$ cup chopped walnuts

$^1/_4$ cup vegan carob (or vegan chocolate chips)

$^1/_2$ cup dried pitted cherries

▸ Place the dates and dried plums into a small saucepan and cover with 1$^1/_2$ cups water. Bring to a boil and simmer for 1 minute, then remove from heat, cover, and let the dried fruit soak while you assemble the rest of the ingredients.

▸ Preheat the oven to 350°F. Spray a 9 x 9-inch baking pan with nonstick spray and set aside.

- Sift or whisk together the barley flour, brown rice flour, carob powder, baking powder, and salt.
- Place the maple syrup, canola oil, vanilla, and the date, dried plum, and water mixture into a blender. Process until completely smooth. Pour the liquid into the dry ingredients and stir together until well combined. Fold in the walnuts, carob chips, and dried cherries.
- Spread the mixture out in the baking pan. Smooth the top using a spatula. Bake for 30 minutes, until the surface springs back to the touch.

FRUIT AND NUT BARS

These bars contain no oil and no sugar; they get their sweetness from dried fruit. They are also chock-full of walnuts, which contain lots of those fabulous omega-3 fatty acids. These bars are wheat- and soy-free—great for those with allergy concerns.

Makes 16 bars

1 cup whole spelt flour

1 cup rolled oats

1/4 cup prune puree (or 1 [2.5-ounce] container baby prunes)

1/2 cup currants (or finely chopped raisins)

1/2 cup dried apricots, finely chopped

1 cup walnuts, chopped

1/3 cup water

- Preheat the oven to 325°F. Lightly coat an 8 x 8-inch pan with nonstick spray and set aside.
- Combine all the ingredients in a large bowl and knead with your hands until a good, stiff dough forms. Add a tablespoon of water if the mixture is too dry. Press dough firmly and evenly into the

prepared pan. Cut into squares with a sharp knife before placing in the oven.

▸ Bake for 25 to 30 minutes, until baked through but still soft (don't overbake them or the bars will be tough). Store leftover bars in the refrigerator.

GINGERBREAD VEGANS

Every year around the Winter Solstice we throw a Gingerbread Cookie Party for all of James's friends. Kids come over to decorate cookies with piping bags of white and colored icing, to drink Silk Nog and sparkling cider, and play games. No gifts are exchanged, but each guest is asked to bring a donation for the local animal shelter. The next day, James and I take the money down to the shelter to wish the animals a happy, homebound holiday.

Makes about 2 to 3 dozen cookies, depending on the size you make them

$1/3$ cup nonhydrogenated margarine, at room temperature

1 cup packed golden brown sugar

1 cup sweet unsulphured molasses

$3/4$ cup water

6 cups all-purpose flour

2 teaspoons baking soda

$3/4$ teaspoon kosher salt

1 teaspoon cinnamon

1 teaspoon ground ginger

$1/2$ teaspoon cloves

$1/2$ teaspoon allspice

For decorating:
Gingerbread Vegan Icing (see page 240)
sprinkles (optional)

- In the bowl of a stand mixer fitted with the paddle attachment, or in a large mixing bowl with a hand mixer, cream together the margarine, brown sugar, molasses, and ½ cup of water.
- In another bowl, sift together the flour, baking soda, salt, cinnamon, ginger, cloves, and allspice. Add the dry ingredients to the wet ingredients, adding just enough of the water to incorporate all the flour and form a dough that holds together well.
- Turn the dough out of the bowl and form into four equal balls. Wrap each ball with plastic wrap and refrigerate for at least 1 hour.
- Preheat the oven to 350°F. Line some baking sheets with parchment paper and spray with nonstick spray. Set aside.
- Working with one ball at a time, roll the dough out on a lightly floured surface with a lightly floured rolling pin. Roll the dough about ¼ inch thick and use cookie cutters to cut out your desired shapes. Use a metal spatula to transfer the cookies to the prepared cookie sheets, placing them about 1 to 2 inches apart.
- Bake for 10 to 12 minutes, until the surface is firm. Transfer to a wire rack to cool completely, then decorate with Gingerbread Vegan Icing (next page).

GINGERBREAD VEGAN ICING

You may want to make multiple batches of this icing and color each with a different food coloring for some very colorful cookie creations. I prefer the look of clean white icing on my little vegans.

Makes about
¾ cup

1 cup sifted powdered sugar

½ teaspoon vanilla

1½ tablespoons Silk Nog or

   1 tablespoon water

Food coloring (optional)

▸ Combine the powdered sugar and vanilla. Sprinkle in the Silk Nog or water, stirring well with a small spatula and using just enough liquid to form a smooth icing. It should be soft enough to squeeze easily out of a piping bag, but not so runny that it runs out of the bag unbidden. Add food coloring, if desired. Transfer the icing to a piping bag fitted with a small round tip and decorate the cookies as desired.

▸ To pack some frosting for the lunch box, put a small amount of icing into one corner of a sandwich-sized resealable plastic bag, then twist the filled corner off and secure snugly with a small rubber band and a piece of holiday ribbon. Cut away the excess plastic at the top of the bag, then cut a very small hole in the tip of the corner to squeeze the icing out. Cover the tip with a bit of plastic wrap so the icing does not dry out before lunch.

HONEYBEE NO-BAKES

These almond-buttery, coconutty no-bake cookies are a favorite of ours all year long, not just at Easter. Roll them into small balls and store in the refrigerator for a quick treat.

Suzanne's Just-Like-Honey is a honey substitute made from brown rice syrup, and it really does taste, well, just like honey! It is available at natural food stores and on the Web. Agave nectar is another vegan honey substitute that is generally available at supermarkets and natural food stores. It is made from the sweet nectar of the agave cactus and is not as thick as honey.

> Makes about
> 33 honeybees

1 $\frac{1}{2}$ cups oat bran

1 cup very finely shredded coconut flakes
   (sweetened or unsweetened, your choice)

$\frac{1}{8}$ cup cocoa powder (or carob powder),
   plus extra for decorating

1 tablespoon vanilla extract

$\frac{1}{4}$ cup almond butter

$\frac{1}{2}$ cup Just-Like-Honey (or agave nectar)

Sliced almonds

▸ For this recipe, the coconut flakes should be very small—just a bit larger than the oat bran flakes. If they are too big, pulse them down to size in a food processor fitted with the S blade.

▸ Line a baking sheet with parchment paper and spray with non-stick spray. Set aside.

▸ In a large mixing bowl, combine the oat bran, coconut, $\frac{1}{8}$ cup cocoa powder, vanilla, almond butter, and liquid sweetener. Knead well with your hands until the mixture holds together.

▸ Pinch off bits of dough (about 2 teaspoons), roll them into ovals, and place them on the baking sheet. Dip your fingers into a bowl of water, if necessary, to keep the dough from sticking.

- Dip a toothpick into the cocoa powder and press two or three lines into the top of each "honeybee" to create stripes. Gently insert an almond slice into each side to resemble wings.
- Store in the refrigerator.

VARIATION: The cocoa stripes are subtle, but cute and all-natural. If you'd like to make yellow stripes instead of brown, mix powdered sugar with powdered yellow food coloring and follow directions above.

NUT AND SEED BUTTER COOKIES

I created this recipe for my friend Mildred and her husband, John, who is gluten-intolerant. They faithfully attended our local vegetarian potlucks since they started—it just wasn't a potluck until Mildred and John came through the door! Unfortunately, they often found themselves with no gluten-free options for dessert, so I made this rich little cookie filled with nut and seed butters especially for them.

Makes 24 cookies

1 cup brown rice flour
1 teaspoon baking powder
3/4 cup natural creamy peanut butter
1/2 cup natural almond butter
1/4 cup raw sesame tahini
3/4 cup pure maple syrup
1 teaspoon vanilla
1/8 teaspoon almond extract
1/4 cup finely chopped toasted unsalted
   sunflower seeds

- Preheat oven to 350°F. Line a baking sheet with parchment paper and set aside.

- In a small mixing bowl, whisk together the brown rice flour and baking powder and set aside.
- In a large mixing bowl, cream together the peanut butter, almond butter, tahini, maple syrup, vanilla, and almond extract with a handheld mixer.
- Add the sunflower seeds and flour mixture and blend until well combined.
- Using your hands, roll the dough into walnut-size balls and place 2 inches apart on the baking sheet (the dough will be oily).
- Flatten the dough balls, using a fork dipped in brown rice flour to make a criss-cross design in the top of each cookie.
- Bake for 18 minutes, or until cookies are golden on the bottom. Remove to a wire rack to cool.

PAXIMADIA COOKIES

These little "Greek biscotti" are lightly sweet and delightfully crunchy. We ate paximadia often at the Greek Orthodox church we attended in California. They are usually flavored with anisette, an anise-flavored liqueur, but I have used alcohol-free anise flavoring here.

Today, most paximadia are made with white flour, but I've taken the recipe back to its roots by using barley flour. For centuries, barley was the staple grain in ancient Greece, and some varieties of paximadia are still made with barley on the island of Crete.

Makes 36 cookies

2 cups barley flour

1 1/2 teaspoons baking powder

1/8 teaspoon kosher salt

1/2 cup nonhydrogenated margarine

3/4 cup sugar

1 teaspoon natural anise flavor (or extract)

¼ cup water

Plain nondairy milk

Raw sesame seeds

▸ Preheat the oven to 350°F. Line a baking sheet with parchment paper and set aside.

▸ In a medium-size mixing bowl, whisk together the barley flour, baking powder, and salt.

▸ In the bowl of a stand mixer fitted with the paddle attachment, cream the margarine and sugar together until light and fluffy (or use a handheld mixer).

▸ Add the anise flavor and beat to combine. Add half the barley mixture, then the water, and then the other half of the barley mixture. Beat until a stiff dough forms.

▸ Turn the dough out onto a smooth surface and knead briefly. Divide the dough in half and form into two long, narrow logs, about 1 inch high, 1½ inches wide, and 9 inches long. Place the logs on the baking sheet. Brush lightly with the nondairy milk, then sprinkle liberally with sesame seeds. Pat the sesame seeds gently into place.

▸ Bake for 35 minutes, until set and golden on the bottom. Remove from the oven and let cool for 15 minutes. Reduce the oven heat to 275°F.

▸ Transfer the logs, one at a time, to a cutting board. Using a very sharp knife, carefully cut the logs into ½-inch slices. Place the slices back on the cookie sheet, cut side down. Bake for 20 minutes, then flip the slices over and bake for another 20 minutes, until slightly dry and golden (they will dry and crisp up more as they cool).

▸ Transfer the cookies to a wire rack to cool completely. Store in an airtight container. Paximadia taste even better the day after they are made.

VEGAN FUDGE

Oooh, this fudge is creamy, rich, smooth, and sweet. Basically, it's everything you ever dreamed chocolate fudge could be. And no one will believe that there's no dairy, butter, or evaporated milk in here. Fudge makes a great holiday gift, too! It can be a bit soft, though, especially if you add the optional marshmallow fluff, so keep it well refrigerated.

Makes one
9 x 9-inch pan,
about 32 pieces

4 cups powdered sugar

1/2 cup cocoa powder

1/2 cup vegan chocolate chips

1/2 cup nondairy milk

2 tablespoons nonhydrogenated margarine

1 1/2 teaspoons vanilla

1 cup cut up vegan marshmallows *or* 1/2 cup vegan marshmallow fluff, like Ricemellow Crème (marshmallows and fluff are optional, but sooo good)

1/2 cup chopped nuts

▶ Spray a 9 x 9-inch baking pan well with nonstick spray and set aside. (For holiday gift giving, I pour the fudge into seven well-sprayed foil baking cups that I buy in the shape of stars, hearts, and so on.)

▶ Sift the powdered sugar and cocoa powder together into a large mixing bowl, add the chocolate chips, and set aside.

▶ In a small saucepan, heat the nondairy milk and margarine to a boil over medium-high heat, stirring constantly to avoid burning.

▶ When the milk is at a steady, strong boil, pour it over the powdered sugar mixture and stir well with a wooden spoon until everything is well combined and the heat has melted the chocolate chips.

▸ Stir in the vanilla, then fold in the marshmallows and the nuts.

▸ Spread the fudge out into the prepared pan(s) and refrigerate for a day or more to solidify.

VARIATION: One inspired test cook used holiday soy nog for the nondairy milk with great results.

Cakes, Puddings, and Desserts

BLACK RICE PUDDING

Black Rice Pudding is a traditional Thai dessert made from chewy wholegrain black rice and creamy coconut milk. This is the best reason James can find for going to a Thai restaurant. He pines and nibbles lightly all through dinner, perhaps deigning to eat one or two morsels of tofu satay, then digs in with gusto when the pudding arrives.

Black rice (also known as "Forbidden Rice") is available at health food stores and Thai markets.

Makes 6 servings

¼ pound raw black rice, rinsed and drained
1 (14-ounce) can light coconut milk
4 tablespoons sugar
A pinch of salt

▸ Place the rice in a 2-quart saucepan. Fill the saucepan with water to within 1½ inches of the top. Bring to a boil, then lower the heat and simmer, partially covered, until the rice is tender, about 30 to 40 minutes. Drain the rice and set aside.

▸ In a small saucepan, bring the coconut milk to a boil. Add the sugar and salt and boil, stirring, for one minute, until sugar dissolves.

▸ To serve, place rice into six dessert cups and top with coconut milk.

▸ Black Rice Pudding is good cold or at room temperature, but it's even better served warm. For lunch, pack the pudding in a lidded container in the lunch box to eat it cold, or pack in a preheated insulated food jar for a luscious hot pudding on a chilly day.

CHOCOLATE BANANA PUDDING

For dessert, prepare this easy, banana-filled pudding the night before. Refrigerate it in a covered lunch container to toss into the lunch box in the morning.

You might want to give carob rice milk a try here. I think carob and banana have a natural affinity; the flavors complement each other quite nicely. Of course, chocolate and banana aren't bad, either!

Makes 4 servings

2 bananas

¼ cup sugar

4 tablespoons cornstarch

2 cups chocolate or carob rice milk
   (or other nondairy chocolate milk)

1 ½ teaspoons vanilla

▸ Slice the bananas into four individual dessert cups or lunch containers. Set aside.

▸ In a medium saucepan, whisk together the sugar and cornstarch. Gradually add the rice milk, whisking constantly. Cook over medium-low heat, stirring constantly with a wooden spoon or whisk, until the mixture comes to a slow bubbling boil. Boil, stirring constantly, for 2 minutes or until thickened.

▸ Remove from heat and stir in the vanilla.

▸ Pour the pudding over the bananas, distributing evenly between the bowls. Refrigerate for several hours or overnight.

CHOCOLATE VEGAN BUTTERCREAM

Makes enough
frosting for
one batch of
Triple Chocolate
Cupcakes
(page 253)

3 cups powdered sugar

1/2 cup cocoa powder

1/2 cup nonhydrogenated margarine

3 1/2–4 tablespoons rice milk

1 1/2 teaspoons vanilla

▸ Sift together the powdered sugar and cocoa powder into a medium-size mixing bowl. Add the margarine, rice milk, and vanilla and beat well using a handheld mixer until the frosting is smooth.

FLUFFY WHITE CUPCAKES

Fantastic, light, fluffy cupcakes—just right for birthdays, classroom parties, or other special occasions.

These taste great with any type of frosting, but I especially like Pineapple Frosting (page 252), which is filled with bits of crushed pineapple.

Makes 22
cupcakes

1 tablespoon apple cider vinegar

1 1/2 scant cups soymilk (plain or vanilla)

2 1/8 cups all-purpose flour

1 1/8 cups sugar

2 teaspoons baking powder

1/2 teaspoon baking soda

1/2 teaspoon kosher salt

1/2 cup canola oil

1 1/4 teaspoons vanilla extract

1/2 teaspoon coconut extract

- Preheat the oven to 350°F. Spray twenty-two muffin cups with nonstick spray or line with paper cupcake liners and spray the liners with nonstick spray. Set aside.
- Place the apple cider vinegar in the bottom of a liquid measuring cup and fill the cup with soymilk to equal 1½ cups. Stir well and set aside (the mixture will curdle).
- In a large mixing bowl, stir together the flour, sugar, baking powder, baking soda, and salt. In another mixing bowl whisk together the soymilk mixture, canola oil, vanilla, and coconut extract. Add the wet to the dry ingredients and beat until smooth using a handheld mixer or stand mixer fitted with the paddle attachment, stopping to scrape down the sides of the bowl.
- Fill each muffin cup with ¼ cup of batter. Bake for 15 to 20 minutes, until a cake tester inserted in the middle of a cupcake comes out clean.
- Let cool in the pans for 5 minutes, then remove the cupcakes from the pan and place them on a wire rack. Let the cupcakes cool completely before frosting with Pineapple Frosting (page 252).

VARIATION: Add sprinkles to the batter before baking for colorful confetti cupcakes.

VARIATION: Visit my website to watch this batter transform into crème-filled, Twinkie-style snack cakes at www.shmooedfood.blogspot.com/2006/01/vegan-twinkies.html. It also makes lovely chocolate-dipped, coconut-covered Australian Lamingtons at www.shmooed food.blogspot.com/2006/05/vegan-lamingtons.html.

GRADUATION HATS

These rich, chocolaty Graduation Hats are made from chocolate cupcakes, graham crackers, and chocolate icing, with fruit leather "tassels." These are a great treat to share with the entire class on its final day. Just don't throw these hats up in the air!

Makes 24 cupcakes

One batch of Triple Chocolate Cupcakes
  (page 253), made without chocolate chips
  and baked without paper liners
24 Chocolate Graham Crackers (page 66),
  baked as 2 1/2 x 2 1/2-inch squares (or use
  store-bought vegan graham crackers)
4 cups powdered sugar
1/2 cup cocoa powder
1/2 cup nondairy milk
2 tablespoons nonhydrogenated margarine
1 1/2 teaspoons vanilla
Several fruit leather strips

▸ Let the cupcakes and crackers cool to room temperature. To make the icing, sift the powdered sugar and cocoa powder together in a medium bowl; set aside.

▸ In a small saucepan, heat the nondairy milk and margarine to a boil over medium-high heat. Transfer to the top of a double boiler or a heat-proof bowl set over a pan of simmering water. Add the powdered sugar mixture and the vanilla. Whisk until completely smooth. Keep the icing over simmering water as you work; the heat will keep the icing soft.

▸ To make the graduation hats, use a sharp, serrated knife to trim off the top of the cupcakes so they sit flat upside down. Dip the bottom and sides of the cupcake into the icing. Set upside down on a wire rack.

▸ Dip a graham cracker square into the icing, covering both sides evenly; use two forks to help turn and coat the cracker. Place the cracker on the top of the upside-down cupcake to form a graduation hat.

▸ To make the tassel, cut fruit leathers into thin strips and arrange on top of the graduation hat before the icing has set.

▸ Let the icing set for about 15 minutes, then transfer to a covered container and keep refrigerated until ready to serve.

PINEAPPLE FROSTING

A quick, easy frosting made with bits of crushed pineapple. This frosting would be perfectly at home on carrot cake, too.

Makes enough frosting for one batch of Fluffy White Cupcakes (page 249).

---

2 cups sifted powdered sugar
1/4 cup nonhydrogenated margarine
1/4 cup well-drained crushed pineapple

▸ Sift the powdered sugar into a medium-size mixing bowl. Add the margarine and crushed pineapple and beat with a handheld mixer. At first, this may seem too dry, but keep beating for about 30 seconds and you will have perfect frosting.

TRIPLE CHOCOLATE CUPCAKES

What would our birthday celebrations be without this recipe? Kids beg for more, while adults swear they're even better than nonvegan chocolate cupcakes. Even omnivorous members of my family ask for this cake for their birthday!

The original version of this recipe was given to me by a woman at a Greek Orthodox church. They must be heaven-sent!

Makes 24 cupcakes or one (9-inch) double layer cake	3 cups all-purpose flour
	1/2 cup cocoa powder
	2 teaspoons baking soda
	1 teaspoon kosher salt
	1 cup sugar
	1 cup packed golden brown sugar
	2 cups water
	1 cup canola oil
	1 tablespoon vanilla
	3/4–1 cup vegan chocolate chips (optional)

▸ Preheat the oven to 350°F. Spray twenty-four muffin cups with nonstick spray or line with paper cupcake liners and spray the liners with nonstick spray. Set aside.

▸ Sift the flour, cocoa powder, baking soda, and salt into a large mixing bowl. Add the sugar and brown sugar, water, canola oil, and vanilla. Mix with a handheld beater or stand mixer until well combined and smooth.

▸ Divide the batter evenly into the twenty-four muffin cups (about 1/4 cup batter in each cup—the cupcakes will rise to fill the muffin cups). Sprinkle the top of each cupcake with some chocolate chips. Bake for 25 to 30 minutes, until a cake tester or toothpick inserted into the middle of a cupcake comes out clean.

▶ Remove from the oven and let cool for about 10 minutes. Transfer the cupcakes to a wire rack to cool completely before frosting with Chocolate Vegan Buttercream (page 249).

VARIATION: To make a cake instead of cupcakes, divide the batter between two 9-inch round cake pans that have been sprayed with nonstick spray. Sprinkle each layer with half the chocolate chips. Bake at 350°F for 40 minutes, until a cake tester or toothpick inserted into the middle comes out clean. Let the cake cool for about 10 minutes, then invert onto a wire rack to cool completely. The frosting recipe makes the perfect amount to frost the cake.

WHEAT-FREE APPLE CRISP

This is my husband's favorite dessert, and he was selfless enough to suffer through several batches while I tested this recipe. I've made it wheat-free so those with wheat allergies can still dig in. It is wonderful served warm from the oven with a glass of vanilla soymilk or soy ice cream, and just as good served cold in a lunch container the next day.

Makes one
9 x 9-inch pan

$3/4$ cup packed golden brown sugar

$2/3$ cup plus 2 tablespoons oat flour

$3/4$ cup quick rolled oats

$1/2$ cup chopped walnuts (or pecans)

$1/4$ teaspoon kosher salt

1 teaspoon cinnamon

$1/2$ teaspoon nutmeg

6 tablespoons canola oil

$2^1/2$ pounds apples, peeled and thinly sliced
    (about 5 apples)

1 tablespoon freshly squeezed lemon juice
2 tablespoons sugar

▸ Preheat the oven to 375°F. Spray a 9 x 9-inch baking pan with nonstick spray and set aside.

▸ To make the topping, mix the brown sugar, oat flour, rolled oats, nuts, salt, cinnamon, and nutmeg together in a large mixing bowl. Add the canola oil and mix well until thoroughly combined. Set aside.

▸ To make the apple filling, toss the sliced apples together with the lemon juice, sugar, and remaining 2 tablespoons oat flour. Put the apple mixture into the baking pan and top evenly with the crisp topping.

▸ Bake for about 1 hour, until the apples are cooked through and the topping is golden brown. Cool on a wire rack before serving.

BEVERAGES

CALCIUM SMOOTHIE

Calcium-fortified nondairy milk, calcium-fortified orange juice, and almonds are all good sources of calcium. Mango gives this smoothie a sweet, tropical taste.

Makes 1 large or
2 smaller servings

- -
$^3/_4$ cup calcium-fortified nondairy milk

$^1/_4$ cup calcium-fortified orange juice

1 tablespoon raw slivered almonds

$^1/_2$ teaspoon vanilla

$^1/_2$ cup frozen mango cubes
- -

▸ Blend all the ingredients in the blender for 1 minute, until smooth. Pack in a juice container with two or three small ice cubes to keep it cold until lunchtime. Give the smoothie a little shake at lunchtime and it's ready to drink.

KID'S ICED TEA

Try this fun alternative to the usual high-calorie, sugary juice drinks. Apple juice ice cubes chill the tea without watering it down, while adding just a hint of sweetness. The ice cubes and tea should be made several hours ahead so they can chill.

Any fruity herbal tea blend will do nicely here. We especially like "Fruit Medley" and "Berry Blues" from Adagio Teas: www.adagio.com.

Makes 1 serving, doubles easily

½ cup organic apple juice

2 tea bags (or 3 heaping teaspoons loose) berry-flavored herbal tea blend

Sugar (optional)

Fresh mint (optional)

▸ Pour the apple juice into an ice cube tray and freeze (make sure the ice cubes will be small enough to fit in your beverage container).

▸ Bring 1½ cups of water to a boil. Place the tea bags in a large mug and pour the hot water in. If using loose tea, place the loose tea in a teapot or French press (plunger pot) and fill with the water. Steep for 10 minutes.

▸ Remove the tea bags. If using loose tea, pour the tea through a strainer. If you wish to add extra sweetener, add 1 teaspoon of sugar to the tea while it is still hot and stir to dissolve.

▸ Place the tea in a well-sealed container (so that it does not pick up other flavors in the refrigerator) and refrigerate for several hours or overnight.

▸ To serve, pour tea into a large glass with apple juice ice cubes. Garnish with a sprig of mint if desired.

WITCHES' BREW

This dark red, sweet, and tangy brew is the perfect drink for your little ghosts and ghouls!

<table>
<tr><td>Makes 1 serving</td><td>1 cup chocolate nondairy milk
½ cup frozen pitted organic sweet cherries</td></tr>
</table>

▸ Combine the chocolate nondairy milk and frozen cherries in a blender and blend until completely smooth. Pack in a beverage container with two ice cubes. Give the brew a little shake at lunchtime, and it is ready to drink.

Recommended Resources

The following lists of books and websites offer cookbooks, guides to proper plant-based nutrition for children, and online resources you may find helpful in packing your own vegan lunch box.

Books

Atlas, Nava. *The Vegetarian Family Cookbook*. New York: Broadway Books, 2004.

Burton, Dreena. *Vive le Vegan! Simple, Delectable Recipes for the Everyday Vegan Family*. Vancouver, British Columbia: Arsenal Pulp Press, 2004.

Davis, Brenda, Bryanna Clark Grogan, and Jo Stepaniak. *Dairy-Free and Delicious*. Summertown, TN: Book Publishing Company, 2001.

Davis, Brenda, and Vesanto Melina. *Becoming Vegan*. Summertown, TN: Book Publishing Company, 2000.

Fuhrman, Joel. *Disease-Proof Your Child: Feeding Kids Right*. New York: St. Martin's Press, 2005.

Lyman, Howard. *No More Bull! The Mad Cowboy Targets America's Worst Enemy: Our Diet*. New York: Scribner, 2005.

Marcus, Erik. *Meat Market: Animals, Ethics, and Money*. Ithaca, NY: Brio Press, 2005.

Moskowitz, Isa Chandra. *Vegan with a Vengeance: Over 150 Delicious, Cheap, Animal-Free Recipes That Rock*. New York: Marlowe & Company, 2005.

Pavlina, Erin. *Raising Vegan Children in a Non-Vegan World*. Las Vegas: VegFamily, 2003.

_____. *Vegan Family Favorites: Tasty and Satisfying Recipes Even Your Kids Will Love*. Las Vegas: VegFamily, 2005.

Pottle, Renee. *The Happy Lunchbox: 4 Weeks of Menus and Recipes*. Kennewick, WA: Hestia's Hearth, 2005.

Stepaniak, Joanne. *The Ultimate Uncheese Cookbook: Delicious Dairy-Free Cheeses and Classic "Uncheese" Dishes*. Summertown, TN: Book Publishing Company, 2003.

Stepaniak, Joanne, and Vesanto Melina. *Raising Vegetarian Children: A Guide to Good Health and Family Harmony*. New York: McGraw-Hill, 2003.

Websites

Bryanna's Vegan Feast: www.bryannaclarkgrogan.com
   Fabulous recipes, resources, and an online newsletter from cookbook author Bryanna Clark Grogan.

Erik's Diner: www.vegan.com
   Erik Marcus, author of *Meat Market and Vegan: The New Ethics of Eating* hosts the first—and still the best—weekly vegan podcast.

Food Fight! Vegan Grocery: www.foodfightgrocery.com
   An online all-vegan grocery store located in Portland, Oregon.

Laptop Lunches: www.laptoplunches.com
   Home of the Laptop Lunch System, the American-style bento box you see pictured in this cookbook.

PETA Kids: www.petakids.com
   PETA has done my son a great service by making veganism look hipper than his frumpy old mom ever could. Their website features in-

formation, quizzes, videos, and games. While you're there, you can sign up for their free magazine, *Grrr!*

Vegan Essentials: www.veganessentials.com

A great shopping site featuring vegan baking supplies, snacks, nutritional yeast, and more.

VegFamily: www.vegfamily.com

Comprehensive resource for raising vegan children, including what to eat during pregnancy, vegan recipes, product reviews, message boards, and more.

Allergen-Free Index

I've included this Allergen-Free Index to help those dealing with allergies or food sensitivities to find recipes they can use. I've discovered that a lot of people with food allergies are drawn to veganism and vegan cookbooks, because by their very nature all vegan recipes contain no dairy products, eggs, fish, or shellfish—some of the most common food allergens. Other common allergens are nuts (including peanuts and tree nuts), soy and soy products, gluten, and wheat. Use the lists here to help you identify recipes free of these foods.

Please also note that many recipes not listed in the index might still be easily modified to suit your needs. For example, peanut butter can be replaced with soy nut butter, chopped nuts can be left out of a muffin recipe, or regular pasta can be replaced with gluten-free rice or quinoa pasta.

Soy-Free Recipes

Gluten-Free Recipes

(Note: may contain oats—look for certified gluten-free oats at your local grocery or health food store)

Wheat-Free Recipes

*All gluten-free recipes above
plus the following:*

Index